GLUTEN-FREE

VEGAN COOKBOOK

FOR BEGINNERS

Over 100 Simple, Delicious and Nutritious Recipe for a Healthier Lifestyle

BONUS: FREE RECIPE JOURNAL FOR PAPERBACK AND HARDCOVER ONLY

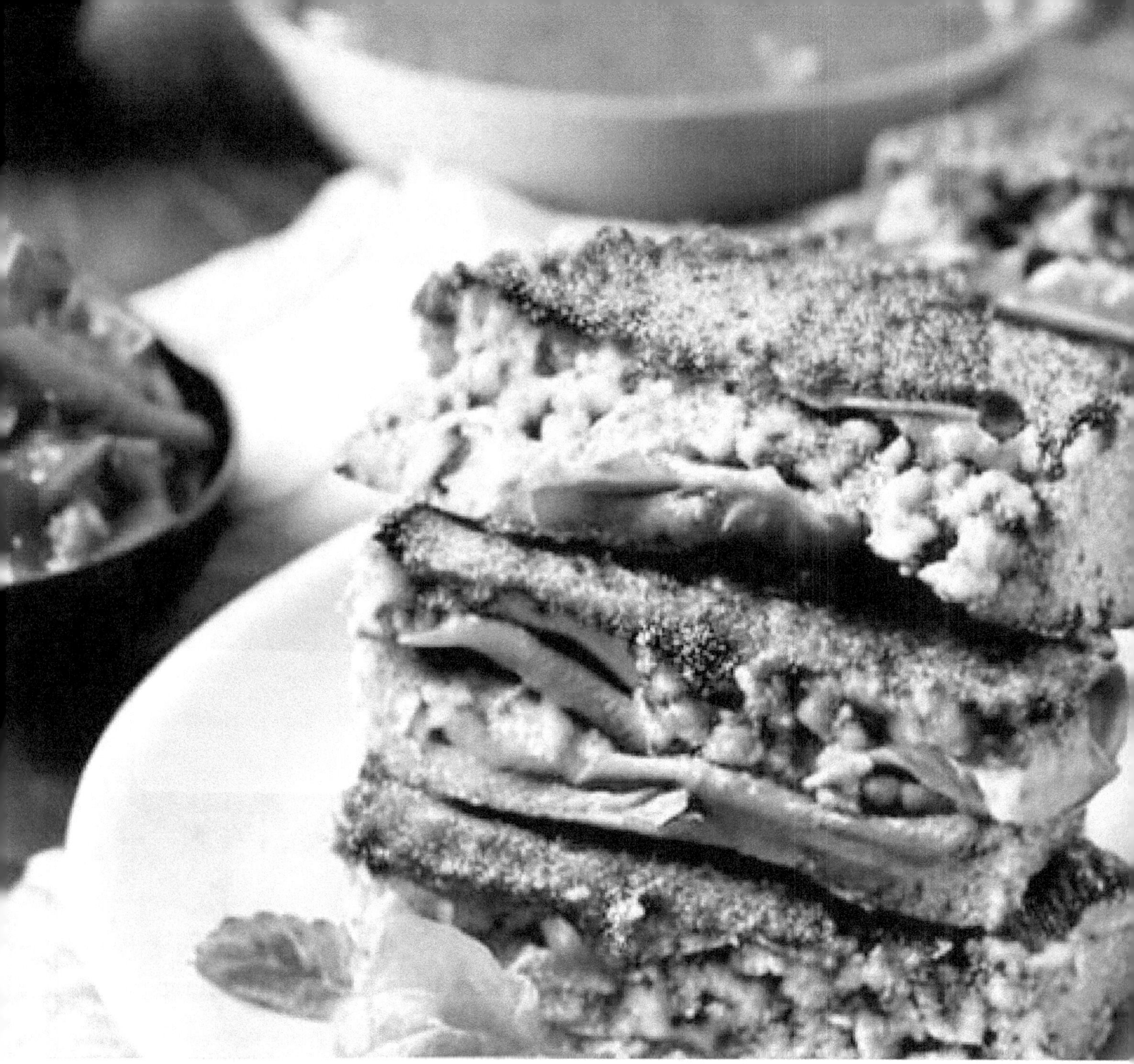

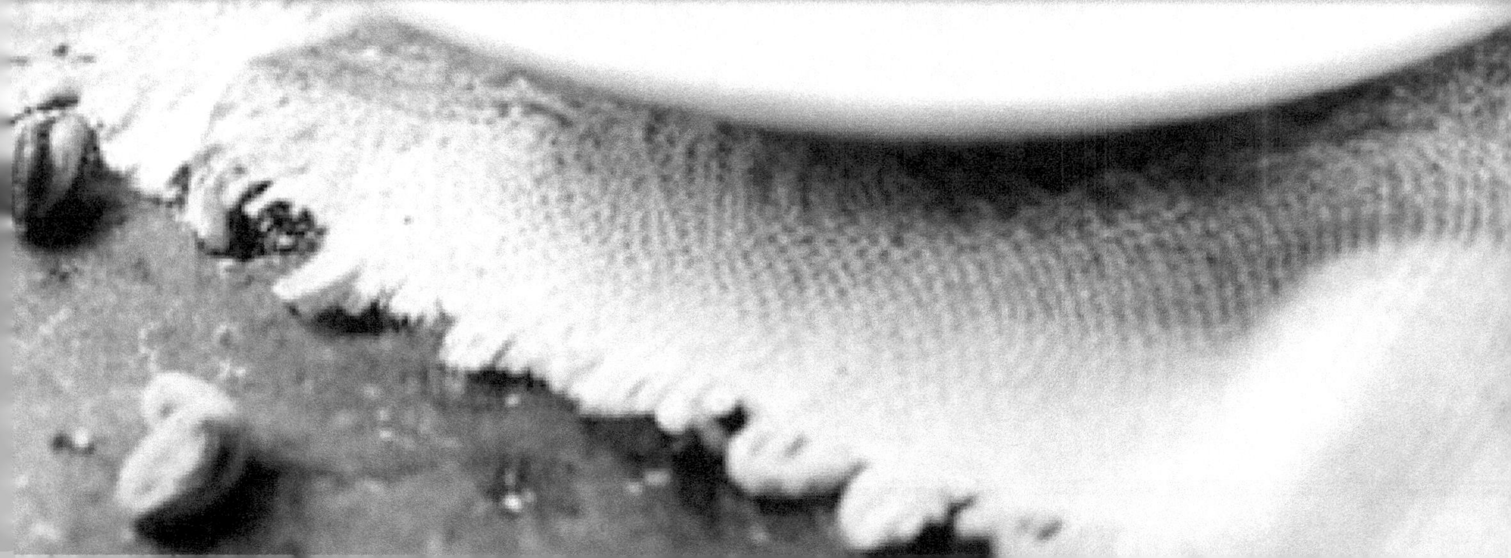

PAULA J. EVANS

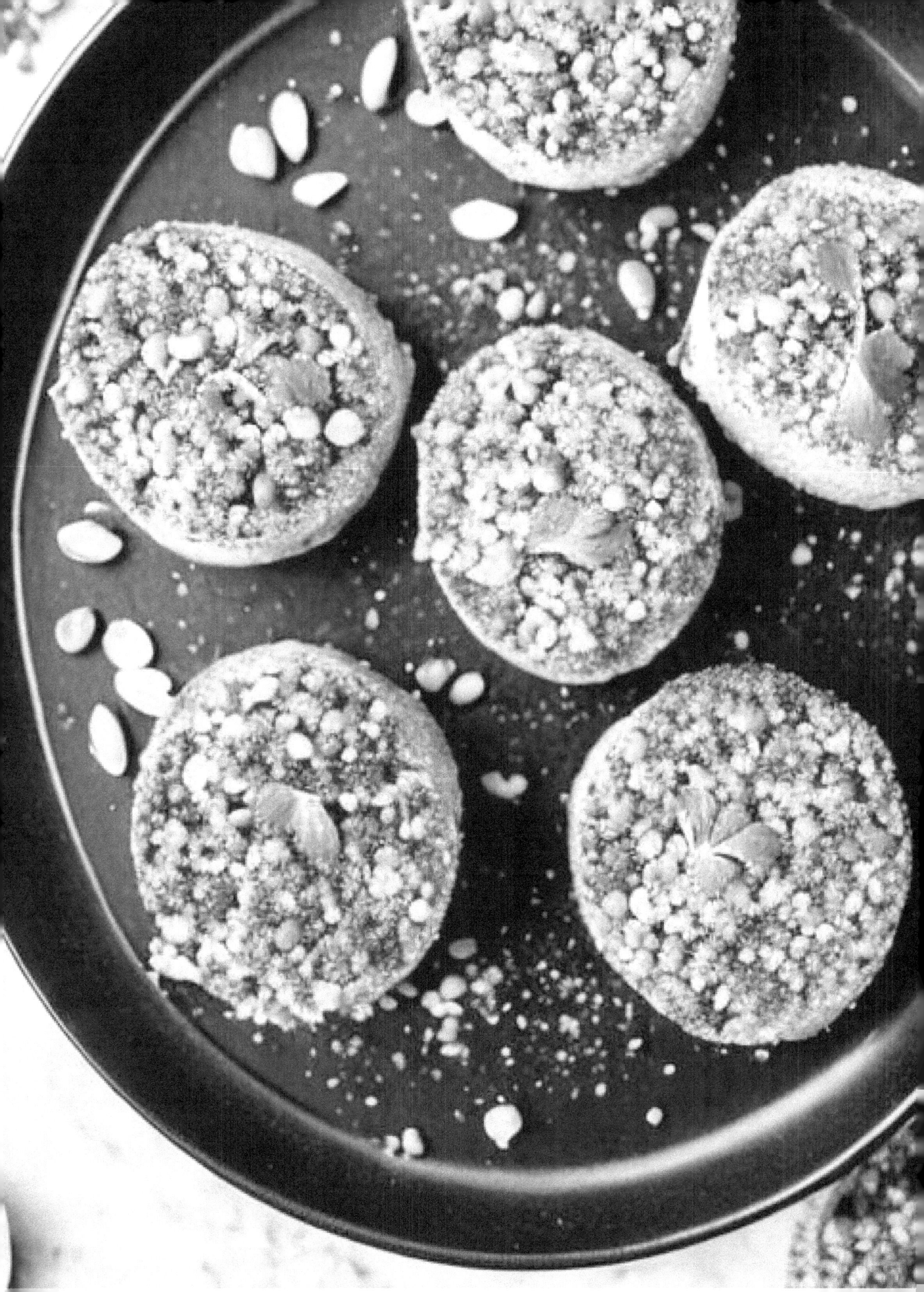

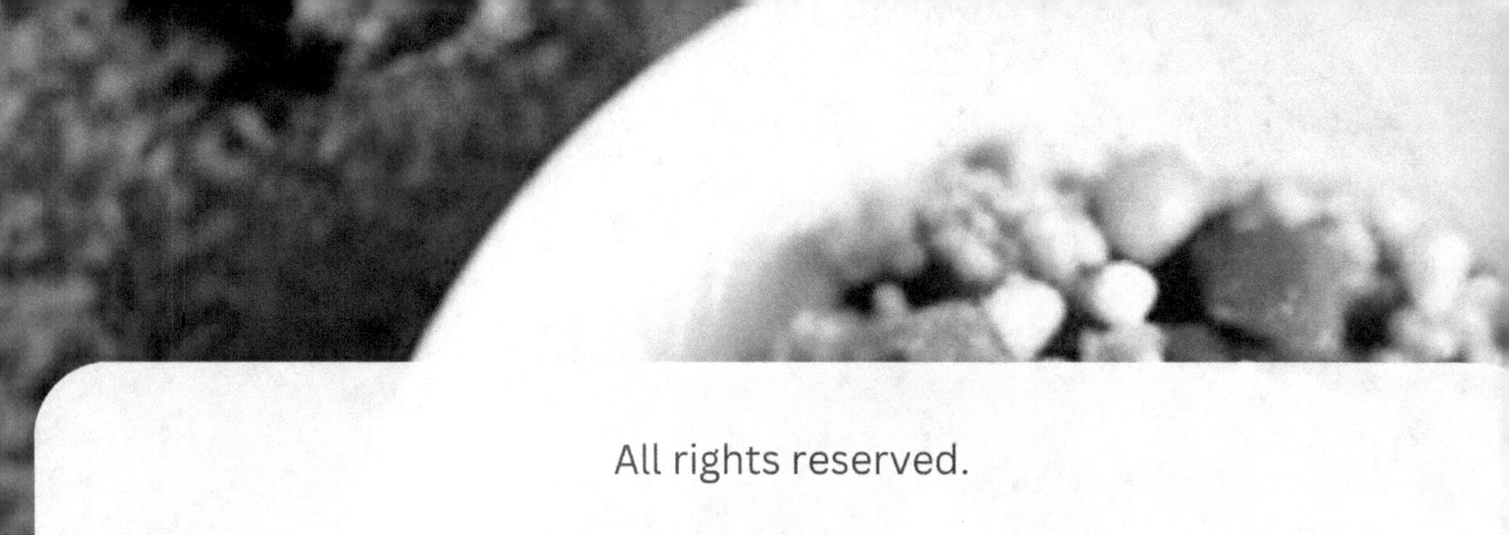

Disclaimer:
The information contained in this book is provided for educational and informational purposes only. It is not intended as a substitute for professional advice, diagnosis, or treatment. Always seek the advice of your physician, therapist, or other qualified healthcare provider with any questions you may have regarding a medical condition or treatment.
The author and publisher of this book have made every effort to ensure the accuracy of the information presented. However, they make no representations or warranties of any kind, express or implied, about the completeness, accuracy, reliability, suitability, or availability with respect to the information, products, services, or related graphics contained in this book for any purpose.

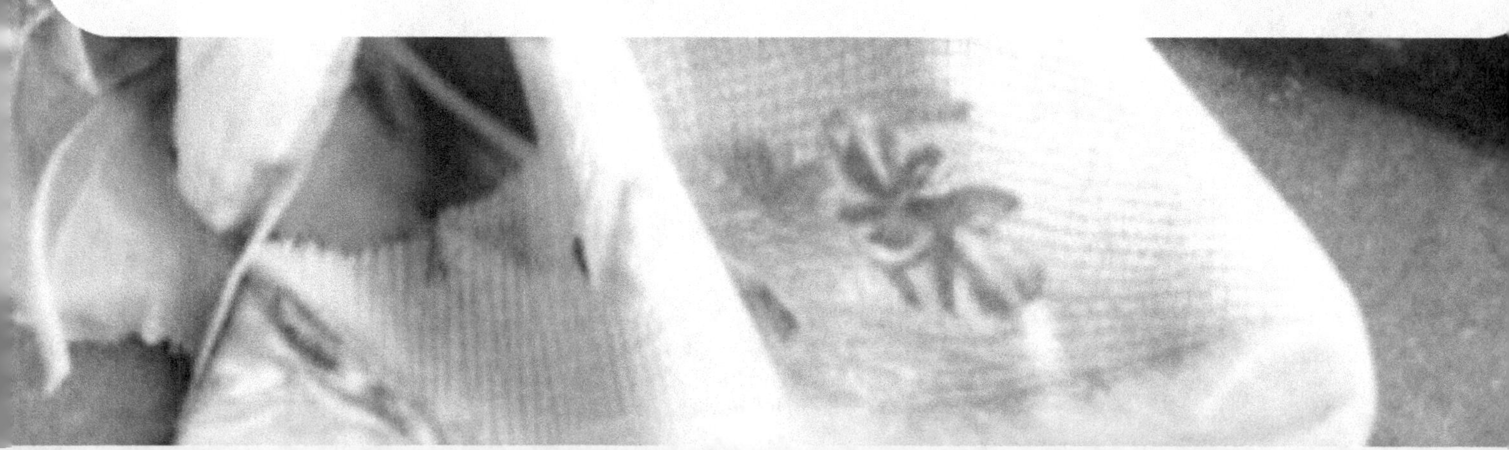

TABLE OF CONTENTS

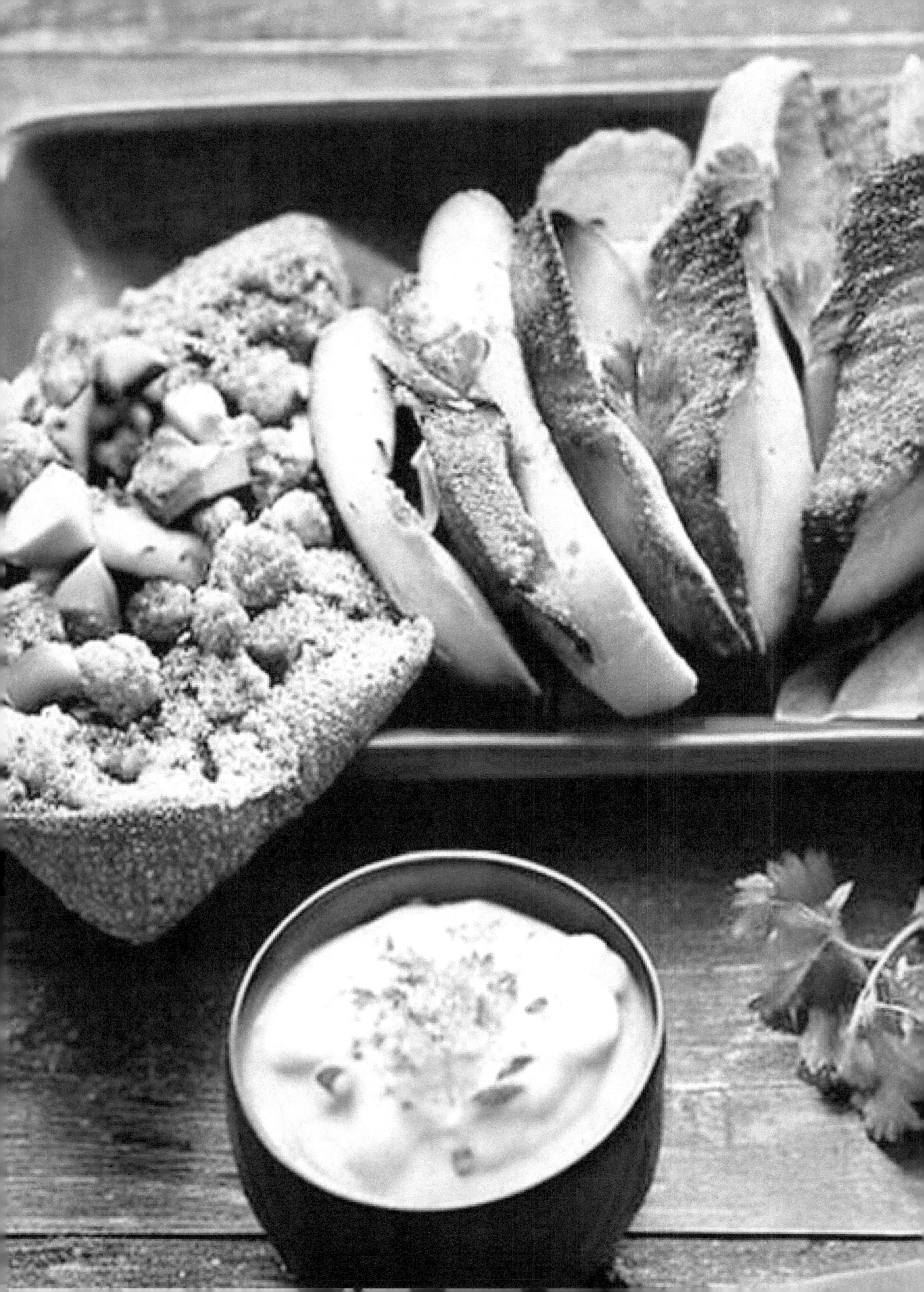

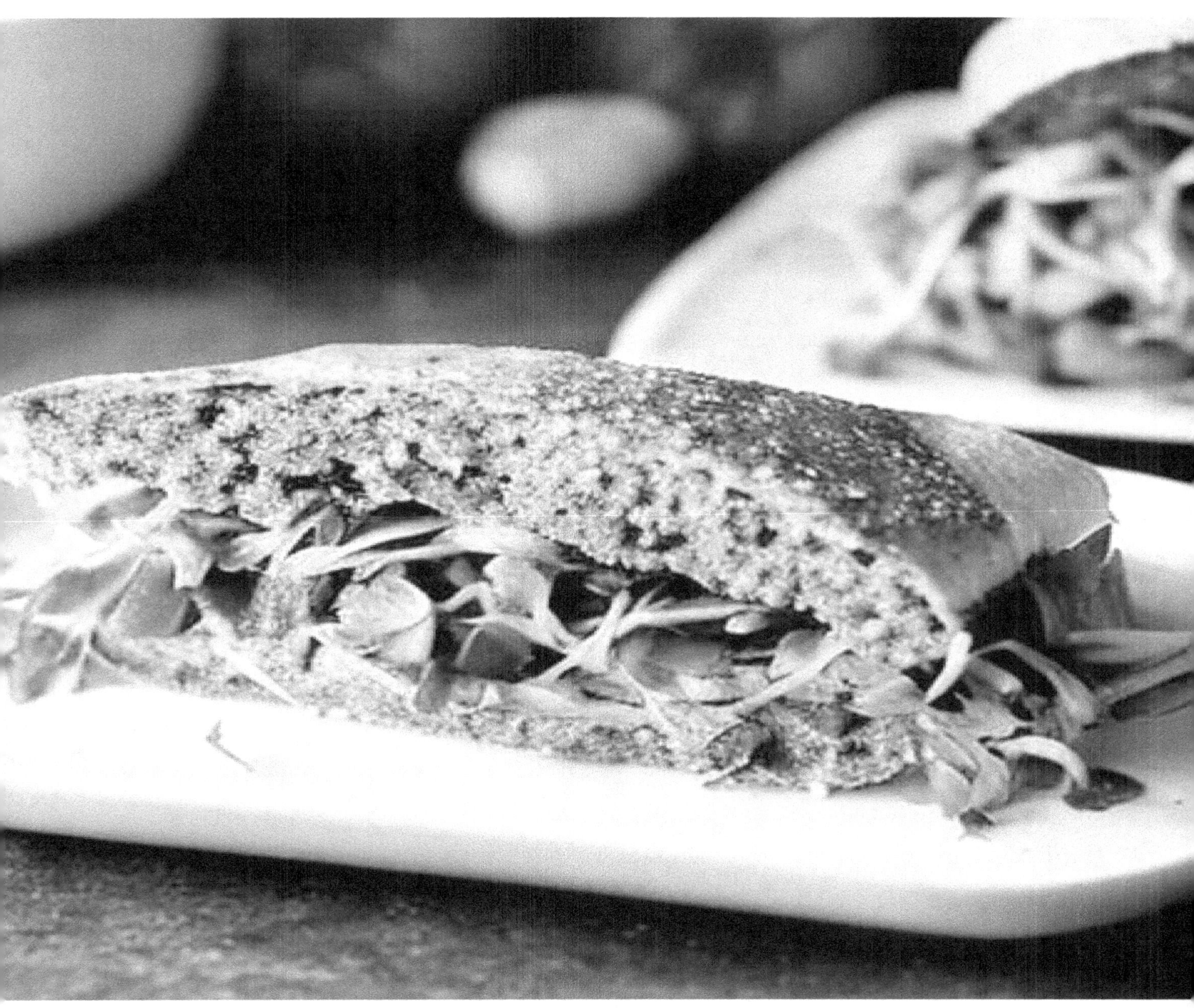

INTRODUCTION

Welcome to The Wonderful World of Gluten-free vegan eating! Some of You May have stumbled upon this book and thought to yourself...gluten-free and vegan? Why both?

In short, this book is intended for people who cannot or choose not to eat animal products or gluten. Some persons get at this type of diet via medical need (like vegetarians who have celiac illness or many allergy issues); others just enjoy cutting down on gluten and animal products because they feel better doing so. This book is not a low-fat book, sugar-free book, or book claiming to save the world. My intention here is to show people how incredibly easy it is to enjoy delicious foods that are 100 percent vegan and gluten-free. I'd like it to be an introduction to this wonderful way of eating for those unfamiliar with this "double diet" and a source of inspiration for all the seasoned gluten free vegan eater sout there. This is a cookbook for vegans, gluten-free folks, and everyone in between

The Gluten-Free Vegan Kitchen

Welcome to the World of gluten-free and vegan cookery. the first step to learning how to cook this manner is to build a grasp of how gluten-free and vegan foods function. This is the most thrilling portion of the book, since you'll discover that a gluten a free and vegan lifestyle doesn't require compromise or sacrifice. Rather, it implies opportunity— opportunity to learn more about food and to discover foods and ingredients that will drastically impact how you think about recipes and your pantry.

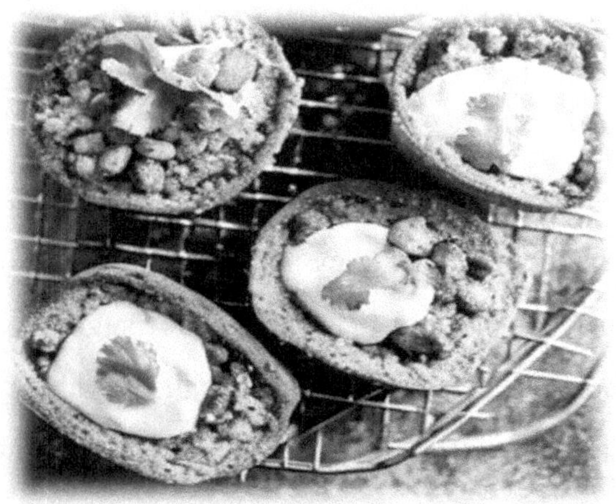

Reasons for Gluten-Free and Vegan

Eating a gluten-free and vegan diet does not imply compromising taste, comfort, heritage, or the pleasure of cuisine. It is obvious from the increased number numerous gluten-free and vegan alternatives at restaurants and supermarkets that there's a market for it, and that people are physically hungry for a variety of meals options. Here are some of the numerous advantages of a gluten-free, vegan lifestyle:

1. **The Heart of Nutrition:** Replacing animal-based goods with plant-based ones drastically decrease your chance for heart disease. Animal products are rich in cholesterol and saturated fats, but vegetables supply a range of vitamins and minerals as well as fiber and phytonutrients.

2. **Pain-Free Movement:** For people with celiac disease or gluten sensitivity, even the slightest quantity of gluten, as little as a crouton, may produce a variety of difficulties that significantly impact comfort, mobility, and their overall sensation of well-being. Cutting down gluten may also decrease the joint discomfort related with inflammation.

3. <u>**Better Complexion:**</u> Gluten and dairy are known to induce an inflammatory reaction that typically causes skin disorders like acne or eczema. Plus, the hormones in dairy may trigger an increase in pore-clogging oil production in your skin. After removing or reducing gluten and dairy, you may observe major changes in your complexion.

4. <u>**Less Water Pollution:**</u> Raising cows for meat or dairy consumes a lot of water. It requires almost 10 times the amount of water to grow an ordinary cow than it does to grow the same weight of grain. Animal husbandry is also a big contributor to water contamination owing to the consequent discharge of animal excrement, antibiotics, and hormones. Going vegan or restricting the usage of animal goods in your lifestyle helps lower your water impact.

5. <u>**Cleaner Eating:**</u> Cooking gluten-free and vegan dishes teaches you to ingredients that are fresh and mainly unprocessed. Most processed foods, unless clearly marked so, include wheat and animal products. When you cook with fresh, natural ingredients, the quality of your meals improves since you're employing higher-quality ingredients.

6. <u>**Increased Energy:**</u> It takes additional energy for your body to digest meat and dairy products. On the other hand, whole foods like fruits, vegetables, and whole grains supply tons of nutrients, give you energy, and keep you feeling fulfilled rather than lethargic and excessively full.

FILL-UP YOUR KITCHEN

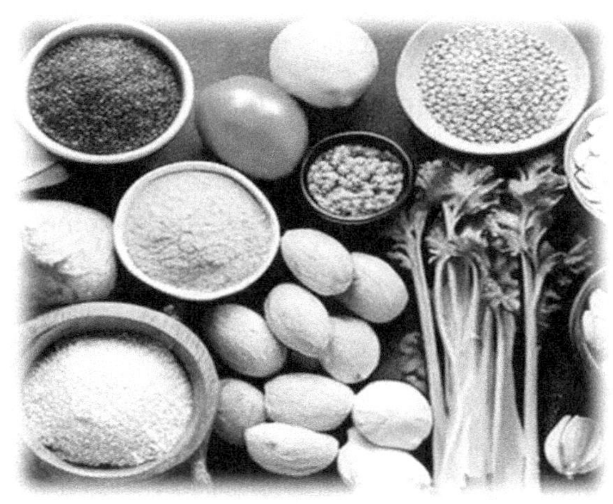

The quality of the meal you produce relies on the components you make it with. But don't panic, it doesn't mean you have to dip into your 401(k) to purchase supplies or seek around the wilderness for morel mushrooms. In this part, you'll learn about the basic, fundamental components of gluten-free, vegan cooking.

It's crucial to understand what gluten is precisely and where it originates from. Gluten is the general term for the proteins contained in wheat, rye, and barley. Those who are gluten intolerant, sensitive, or allergic are impacted by the prolmins, or proteins, in these cereals. These proteins are what provides wheat based items on their form, chew, and stretchy feel. Gluten-free flours do not contain these proteins, hence they are commonly combined with other nutrients like xanthan gum, agar, and starches in recipes to generate a similar outcome. Throughout this book you will use a range of gluten-free flours for breads, batters, and cakes. Here are some of my favorites:

GLUTEN-FREE ALL-PURPOSE BLENDS

These blends are frequently a combination of rice flours, starches, sorghum, and a gum or binder like xanthan. Every brand has its own versions, with varied results. I normally use my own mix (here) since it's simple to produce and inexpensive, and it offers me the most consistent results. You will be utilizing gluten-free all-purpose flour repeatedly throughout this book, and a five-pound the package will get you through most of the recipes. If you prefer to purchase it prepared,

I prefer Bob's Red Mill Gluten-Free 1 to 1 Baking Flour or King Arthur Baking Company's Gluten-Free Measure for Measure Flour.

OAT FLOUR

Oats on their own are gluten-free, since they do not contain the prolamins that provoke gluten allergies and sensitivities. Nonetheless, oats are commonly cultivated close to wheat and rye or processed using the same machinery, leading to cross-contamination. Look for the gluten-free label on oat flour or oats if you have a gluten intolerance. Oat flour is moderate in taste and produces an airy texture to pancakes and waffles.

OTHER FLOURS

Almond flour has become a popular gluten-free choice since it contains a small nutty taste and delivers the same nutritional advantages as eating almonds; nonetheless, it may be thick and bit gritty, so always be sure to use finely ground flour. Coconut flour is gluten-free, low carb, and low calorie. However, it may also be incredibly thick, and, well, it tastes like coconut. You should utilize around 75 percent less coconut flour than the quantity of all-purpose flour called for in a recipe. Both almond and coconut flours should be mixed with another flour to lessen their consistencies and flavors. Despite its name, buckwheat flour is not part of the wheat family and does not include gluten. It adds its nutty aroma to baked foods, however it does not supply structure; you'll need to add stabilizers like xanthan gum or starch to hold buckwheat breads and other delights together.

2. Dairy Alternatives

The range of viable dairy replacements has quickly grown in the past recent years as more individuals have found the dietary and health advantages of removing dairy from their diets. Dairy has large quantities of saturated fats and hormones that contribute to a number of health issues. Below are a few dairy replacements for gluten-free and vegan recipes. If you'd want to produce your own nondairy milk, click here in the Basics chapter.

COCONUT MILK

There are two primary varieties of coconut milk that you may get in stores:

Canned and Packaged. Canned coconut milk, mainly found in the international part of the market, is thicker and includes more fat than the packaged variety that's available on the health food stores. Canned coconut milk is marked according to the quantity of natural fat and sweetness it contains.

Choosing a type depends on the recipe. Baked items may employ the packed manner, but desserts and curry sauces benefit from the additional fat in the can for texture and taste.

ALMOND MILK

Almond milk is available both in the refrigerated section and on shelves in the health food sections in supermarket shops. The chilled version is frequently thicker and has less preservatives, although both may be used for baked goods. Almond milk is not suggested for savory sauces because of the modest inherent sweetness that may be off-putting in savory meals.

OAT MILK

Oat milk has gained popularity in recent years, due to coffee shop baristas. Its thick texture and ability to produce foam makes it a fantastic option for lattes and other coffee beverages. It is also the best nondairy, gluten-free milk for savory recipes due of its neutral flavor and thick consistency. If you're sensitive to gluten, it's crucial to check oat milk labels for cross-contamination or build your own (see here).

3. Oils and Fats

Fat is a vital macronutrient that supports with digestion, brain health, and vitamin absorption. There are several vegan oils and fats that are fantastic for baking, and many popular brands like Country Crock now offer nondairy butters. When baking, fat is necessary for stability, light texture, and color.

VEGAN BUTTER

Non Dairy butter has taken over the store aisles, with several brands supplying baking sticks, spreads, and even European-style cultured butters. The most popular brand of vegan butter is Earth Balance, which generates both soy-based and vegetable oil variants. Each vegan butter is slightly varied in taste and price range, but all work well for baking and sautéing.

COCONUT OIL

Pure coconut oil, not virgin, is prevalent in many recipes because of its high fat content. Butter is normally approximately 65 percent saturated fat, but coconut oil is 90 percent saturated fat. This high fat content has both advantages and cons. Coconut oil is solid at ambient temperature, which makes it suitable for raw delicacies like vegan cheesecake. On the other side, however, the high fat content also makes it one of the least healthful oils.

OLIVE OIL

Olive oil is one of the most regularly used oils, and it comes with nutritious antioxidants. This oil is prepared by crushing olives without much additional processing. Extra-virgin olive oil offers the highest taste and health advantages, as it is not heat treated and originates from the initial pressing of the olives. An excellent bottle of extra-virgin olive oil will arrive in a dark glass bottle or box, will taste strong and a touch bitter like fresh olives, and will have a "best by" date printed on the box. Rancid or poor-quality olive oil could smell like walnuts and have touches of a crayon-like flavor.

NEUTRAL OILS

Grapeseed, peanut, maize, and vegetable oils are the finest for frying because of them high smoke points and lack of taste. Grapeseed oil is prepared utilizing a natural processing technique and is strong in omega-6 fatty acids, which makes it a more heart-healthy alternative than butter, shortening, or coconut oil. Grapeseed oil may be pricey, but its neutral flavor permits additional substances like herbs and spices shine.

4. Starches and Gums

When you bake without gluten, you need starches and gums to offer stability and texture to your breads, pastries, and other baked goods; gluten-free flours such almond, sorghum, and coconut do not have the ability on their own to produce cohesion, so the starches and gums offer flexibility and chew. Gums and starches each have their own specialized application, dependent on the sort of recipe and desired final result.

XANTHAN GUM

Xanthan gum is used in gluten-free goods because it resembles the structure of gluten for baked foods. It is made by fermenting sugar with the bacterium Xanthomonas campestris and then drying and powdering the thick paste. It is extensively used since it is simple to manufacture, allergen-free, flavorless, and odorless.

TAPIOCA STARCH

Tapioca starch is sold in supermarkets under a number of names, such as tapioca flour and cassava flour. This popular thickening may be changed in for cornstarch with virtually comparable results. The advantage of utilizing tapioca starch above other forms of starch is that it keeps its thickening qualities for a longer heating duration. It also provides a subtle gloss to sauces.

CORN-STARCH

Cornstarch is the most frequent thickening and the most cost friendly of the starches. However, it is heavy in calories and carbs with little nutritional advantage.

5. Pasta and Grains

Pastas and grains provide the base for many of the main dish dinners because they add bulk, texture, taste, and nourishment. The recipes in this book includes several different gluten-free grains to offer a diverse range of unusual flavors and sensations.

GLUTEN-FREE PASTA

The number of accessible gluten-free pastas has increased in recent years. You may now obtain protein-rich chickpea flour, fiber-rich lentil pasta, and especially low-carb konjac or shirataki noodles (Japanese noodles manufactured from the konjac plant). The biggest danger of using gluten-free noodles is that they do not cook the same as wheat-based versions, therefore follow the packaging instructions attentively.

RICE

Rice is often used as a basis for dishes since it is easy to prepare, inexpensive, simple to purchase in any food shop, and shelf stable. Different cuisines employ various varieties of rice according on taste, ethnic heritage, or cooking time; however, kinds of rice may often be switched depending on desire or availability. When picking a kind of rice, consider a few things: flavor, consistency, fragrance, and nourishment. Basmati, a long-grain rice used in Indian meals, is very fragrant and low on the glycemic index (which reflects how fast your body absorbs the nutrients and, hence, how much it surges your blood glucose levels. Lower is normally preferable). Sushi rice, a brief grain is highly sticky and is the highest on the glycemic index. Brown rice types are the least processed, provide the highest insoluble fiber and phytonutrients, and tend to be chewier. Recipes in this book will commonly call requires a specific sort of rice, but feel free to substitute in your preferred variety and alter the cooking times as required.

POLENTA/GRITS

Polenta (a.k.a. grits) is created from dried and powdered maize, although it is coarser than cornmeal. When cooked, polenta makes a thick porridge that is a fantastic basis for a stew, marinara sauce, or roasted vegetables. When chilled, you can use it to produce a cake that can be cut and then fried, baked, or grilled.

QUINOA

Quinoa, which is essentially a seed, is one of the most well-known wholesome foods that may be purchased in any grocery shop. It's so popular because it includes all nine necessary amino acids, is rich in protein and fiber, and includes loads of vitamins and minerals. It has a somewhat crunchy feel when prepared and is used extensively throughout this text. Be careful to rinse your quinoa before using if the product isn't branded "pre-rinsed."

OTHER GRAINS

Gluten-free grain choices have grown increasingly available as food firms race to feed the growing demand. Each grain delivers various flavors and textures, and some even have a quick cooking time. Buckwheat groats are nutty, big, and extremely chewy, which makes for a terrific hot morning cereal. Millet is a small grain with a quick cook time and is comparable in texture to couscous. Sorghum, a blooming plant, features pearl-like grains that make for a wonderful cold grain and vegetable salad. These grains are typically marketed in the same region as wheat grains, thus it is vital to check for the gluten-free Label.

6. Other Pantry Items

A well-stocked pantry is crucial to ensure that home-cooked meals happen. You don't need to have a doomsday bunker ready, but it's prudent to get some affordable pantry staples in bulk.

BEANS

Beans, either dry or canned, provide a convenient protein source for a number of meals. The most frequent beans used throughout this book are black beans, pinto, kidney, and cannellini. Dried beans can be kept longer and are less processed, but they need extended boiling periods. Canned beans are the simplest choice but may potentially add a lot of salt to dishes.

LEGUMES

Legumes are the seeds of the Fabaceae plant family and include black-eyed peas, chickpeas, peanuts, and lentils. Legumes are rich in fiber and protein and are widespread in both gluten-free and vegan diets. Beans and legumes are typically used interchangeably in recipes; however, some individuals exclude legumes from their meals due of probable inflammatory consequences.

NUTS

Nuts, both raw and roasted, are prevalent in vegan cookery since they are abundant in natural lipids and protein. Keep a range of them on hand, including cashews, peanuts, and walnuts, for recipes and nutritious snacks. If you have a nut allergy, there are numerous seeds that may be used in lieu of nuts, such sunflower, pumpkin, and sesame seeds. Be careful to acquire the raw versions of nuts and seeds if you wish to cream them.

7. Seasonings

Your spice cabinet is one of the most crucial pieces of your kitchen because with the correct ingredients, you can create just about any taste. Also, investing a little extra on fresh, high-quality spices guarantees that you're the food will have the greatest taste and the nicest scent imaginable.

SALT

Kosher salt is used for several of this book's recipes and will be designated specifically. It's a bigger grain, which implies less salt by volume while still being plenty salty. Be cautious if you switch salts, since a finer-grain salt will yield a much saltier meal. Stock your cupboard with table salt, kosher salt, and flaked salt for a final touch to a dessert or dinner.

GLUTEN-FREE TAMARI AND COCONUT AMINOS

Soy sauce includes gluten, but thankfully there are two wonderful subs: gluten-free tamari and coconut aminos. These are both wonderful ingredients for soups, stews, and tofu. They both add salty, savory, umami taste to a range of dishes.

NUTRITIONAL YEAST

Nutritional yeast, or as the hip vegans call it, "nooch," is an ingredient to stock up on when you get into vegan cookery. It has a nice cheesy flavor, and it's used to add umami to dishes and as a topping in lieu of Parmesan. Plus, it is an excellent source of B vitamins.

SPICES AND HERBS

Having a broad choice of tastes on available provides you alternatives to create a dish. You'll see a number of these herbs and spices throughout the book:

• Basil

• Chili powder

• Ground coriander

• Ground cumin

• Garlic and onion powder

• Ground ginger

• Ground mustard

• Oregano

• Paprika and smoked paprika

Reading Labels

Checking product labels to confirm that they meet both vegan and gluten-free criteria might seem like a difficult undertaking. However, there are a few suggestions and methods to make grocery shopping a breeze. Buying items that are themselves ingredients, rather than goods that include ingredients, is a straightforward approach to know precisely what you're receiving. But sometimes it's good to like the convenience of prepared dishes, rather than creating each component of a recipe from scratch. There are certain crucial elements to remember when deciding whether a product is fit for your lifestyle. All goods that contain or may include known allergies must be marked with allergen declarations. The "may contain" disclaimer is used, for example, when an otherwise gluten-free food is produced or processed in the same facility as items that do contain gluten therefore there is a possibility of cross-contamination. Products tagged "may contain gluten" are okay for those on low-gluten diets who are not allergic to gluten, however they are not safe for persons who develop severe responses to gluten.

Vegan Labelling

Animal-derived components represent about half of the eight main food allergies. This implies that items that include eggs, fish, shellfish, and milk must, by law, be properly stated as such on food packaging. Other non-vegan components may be a bit sneakier. Look out for the obvious culprits including steak, poultry, and honey. More inconspicuous non vegan components include gelatin, carmine, and L-cysteine. The phrase "natural flavors" may also mask a variety of animal products, including as castoreum, a food ingredient produced from beaver glands that is widely used to imitate vanilla taste.

The good news is that there are several applications accessible It enables you to scan a product and take away the guesswork. PETA.org, for instance, really verifies with the food businesses themselves to ascertain whether there are animal products under the broad phrase "natural flavors." There are also a number of vegan-certified labels that you can look out for, such as "Vegan Certified" and "Plant-Based."

Gluten-Free Labelling

Gluten is a bit simpler to detect in an ingredient list than animal products are. As a significant allergy, wheat should always be specified in the allergen statement the product packaging, even if the product only contains traces. Gluten-free goods may also be clearly recognized by a "GF" mark or "GFCO," which stands for the Gluten-Free Certification Organization.

SNEAKY NON-VEGAN FOODS

Being a vegan supermarket shopper means you need to be an ingredient list super detective. Often a product is accidently vegan, therefore isn't branded as such, like most ketchups, Cracker Jack Caramel Coated Popcorn, and classic Pringles. However, many other dietary items have

Hidden elements that make them not vegan friendly, such as:

- **<u>Marshmallows:</u>** Gelatin is the enemy of vegans since it is in so many foods. marshmallows nearly generally include gelatin, save for vegan ones like dandies.
- **<u>Granola bars:</u>** Granola bars frequently sneak in non-vegan ingredients like honey and whey. Most Clif Bars and Kashi granola bars are unintentionally vegan, however, and all of the LÄRABAR original fruit and nut bars and Go Macro Macro Bars are vegan.
- **<u>Kimchi:</u>** It is crucial to examine the label of this wonderful, spicy Korean

pickle because fish paste or fish sauce is commonly used.

- **Collagen:** This ubiquitous beauty product and processed food ingredient may be manufactured to be vegan friendly, although, unless it is clearly indicated, collagen is predominantly created from animal-based ingredients.

- **Food coloring:** Some hues are plant-derived, whereas others, like Natural Red #4, is created employing carmine, which comes from crushed beetles. Your best chance is to avoid any goods that use food coloring or use only foods with the Certified Vegan label.

- **Cereal:** Many popular cereals should be vegan based on the ingredients list. Yet, many enriched grains include vitamin D3 which is created from sheep's lanolin.

- **Confectioner's glaze (a.k.a. shellac):** Most sweets and sprinkles utilize confectioner's glaze in order to attain that polished end result. Shellac is created up of crushed bugs and may also be termed food glaze or natural glaze.

- **Casein:** Casein, the primary protein in dairy milk, is typically disguised in the ingredient lists because goods that are branded "dairy-free." Whenever you buy creamy soup, ice cream, sorbet, or pudding mix, watch out for this deceptive addition.

- **Salt and vinegar chips:** There are both vegan and non-vegan variants of lactic acid discovered in salt and vinegar chips. Whey is in the non-vegan version. Most salt and vinegar chips include the non-vegan variant, so check the label.

- **Bread:** Whey crops up in most store-bought breads. Companies typically will write "contains whey" at the end of the ingredients list.

Gluten is classified as a significant allergy, which implies that gluten should be declared on product labels and ingredient listings. However, if you're sensitive to gluten or encounter severe symptoms Regarding gluten, pay extra attention to the ingredient labels when you buy any of these products:

- **Candy:** Malt or malt extract, produced from barley (which includes gluten), are typically included to candies and chocolates as a sweetener.

- **Soy sauce:** Soy sauce includes wheat and/or utilizes malt flavoring.

- **Beer:** A variety of gluten-containing grains is utilized to manufacture beer in the mash stage. There are certified gluten-free beer alternatives.

- **Bottled salad dressing:** Many salad dressings include hidden sources of gluten, and some even contain subtle non-vegan components. Malt vinegar is the major gluten-containing cause, but also watch out for Worcestershire sauce and anchovies in Caesar dressing (both are obviously not vegan).

- **Seitan and other vegan meats:** Seitan, which is a popular vegan protein source, is created completely of wheat gluten.

- **Rolled oats:** Oats on their own are gluten-free; nonetheless, they commonly become cross-contaminated with gluten if they are cultivated in a field with or processed in the same facility as wheat and rye. Gluten-free oats are prominently marked and generally have a different color top than oats that may contain gluten.

- **Flavored potato chips:** Malt vinegar and wheat flour are prominent flavor enhancers for potato chips. Soy sauce is also occasionally used to season potato chips.

- **Bouillon cubes:** Bouillon cubes and other spice mixes typically include malt dextrin, which may be generated from wheat. There are gluten-free choices available, however it is much simpler to create your own stock from leftover vegetable scraps (see here).

- **Dried fruit:** Dried fruit on its own is gluten-free, although it commonly becomes cross-contaminated on processing equipment. If you have a gluten sensitivity, it is crucial to choose dried fruit that is branded gluten-free.

- **Soup:** Cream-based or creamy alternatives like tomato soup are typically prepared using wheat as a thickener in the roux step. There are gluten-free choices available, and they will be clearly marked.

Essential Tools and Equipment

These basic products can make your culinary experience smoother and more fun:

1. **Metal measuring spoons and cups:** Spending the little bit more for metal measuring tools is a smart long-term investment since they won't warp could crack from usage.

2. **Baking pans:** Large rimmed baking sheets (a.k.a. half sheet pans) enable

you to bake and roast without the danger of your ingredients falling over into your oven, and it's worth having more than one. A 12-mould muffin The pan may be used for both muffins and cupcakes.

3. **Whisks:** Having at least two whisks saves you the effort of washing one while you're in the midst of cooking. I suggest a balloon whisk, which is big and bulbous, and a thin French whisk, which is useful for smaller quantities or bowls.

4. **Wooden spoons and rubber spatulas:** A thick wooden spoon (I prefer one with a little heaviness) is ideal for creating stews, doughs, and sauces. You'll also need a couple of rubber spatulas of varied sizes.

5. **Tongs:** Tongs are either totally metal or equipped with high-heat silicone ends. I like the silicone-tipped tongs since they assure that you won't scratch your kitchenware.

6. **Potato masher:** You'll need this item to crush beans, break down fruits for jams and sauces, and, yes, mash potatoes.

7. **Knives:** A nice chef's knife is an investment that can speed up your prep job and help you prevent kitchen catastrophes. The sharper the knife, the less likely you are to slip when cutting slippery foods. A tiny santoku knife is my go-to for most chopping, but I also use my paring knife regularly for cutting or destemming fruit.

8. **Pots and pans:** It goes without saying that pots and pans are vital kitchen products, but here is actually where you should spend your kitchen money. The decision is yours between ceramic lined, nonstick, high-quality stainless steel, or cast iron. The general guideline is that the heavier the pot or pan, the better it will be at heat distribution and lifespan. I prefer nonstick pans since they enable me to avoid extra oil, but I also use stainless steel pots so I don't have to worry about damaging the coating while mashing or using my immersion blender. I also have a few good seasoned cast iron pots for blackening vegetables.

9. **Food processor:** Use this kitchen workhorse to cut vegetables, break down nuts and grains, pulse cold butter into flour, then blend beans and vegetables for dips.

10. **Immersion blender:** You may acquire a high-quality immersion blender for roughly $25, and you'll use

it regularly for pureeing soups and preparing sauces.

Nice-to-Have Tools and Equipment

The more you cook, the more conscious you'll become of the exciting and new kitchen devices that may make cooking and prep simpler. There are numerous kitchen gadgets that are worth the cost, however before you acquire the newest and flashiest thing, conduct a little study to discover if there's additional equipment that may do a multitude of jobs rather than a single activity.

- **Rice cooker:** A rice cooker may be used for much more than simply rice. I use it can cook grains, oats, risotto, and even soup without the concern of burning or the difficulty of stirring.
- **High-speed blender:** A high-speed blender might have a heavy price tag, which makes it more of a desire than a necessity. However, paying more upfront on a high-quality blender means fewer replacements and repairs later.
- **Pressure cooker:** A pressure cooker may speed up cooking times and make meal prep is easy.
- **Air fryer:** This tiny, fast-cooking equipment simulates frying with little to no oil.

Ways to Make Gluten-Free and Vegan Work

If you are new to cooking without gluten and animal-based foods, the procedure could seem a little intimidating, but it doesn't have to be. Here are eight ideas and tactics to make gluten-free and vegan cooking not merely accessible yet interesting and easy:

- **Cook without borders:** Certain foreign cuisines tend to need less gluten and less animal-derived substances than others. Think Indian curries, Thai stir-fries, and Spanish paella. Travel the globe without leaving the coziness of your kitchen.
- **Meal plan like a pro:** Ever heard the old proverb, "Failing to plan is planning to fail"? Whether it requires organizing out your meals for the week or batch cooking so you've always have a well-stocked freezer, meal planning helps lessen the stress of not knowing what to eat.
- **Shop with a list:** Don't forget to jot down precise brand names, particularly if you share shopping duties with other members in your family; This will avoid misunderstanding and decrease time spent reading labels.

- **Embrace the potluck:** Food intolerances and lifestyle choices don't imply you can't get sociable! Potlucks are a terrific way to celebrate since you know sure what you're carrying is suited for your lifestyle.
-
- **Become the master of packed snacks:** Whether you're on a road trip or during a long day at the office, fast, handy snacks are vital. Pack homemade trail mix, crispy chickpeas, roasted seaweed, and homemade granola bars.
- **Take the vitamins:** If you're getting enough calories from diverse sources, chances are you're receiving most of the vitamins and minerals you need. However, there are certain necessary minerals, such as B12

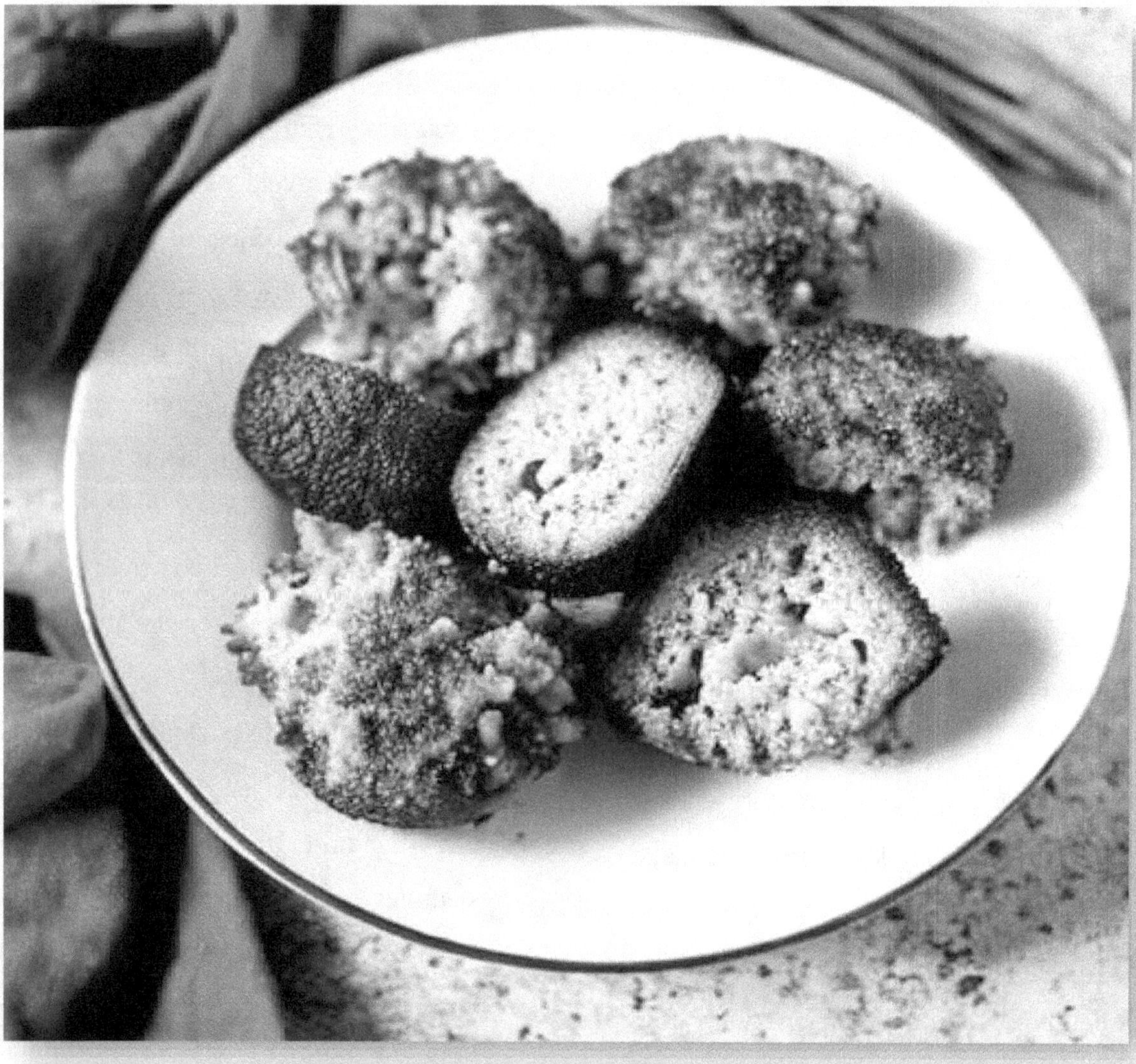

CHICKPEA FLOUR OMELET

- Prep time: 5 minutes
- Cooking time: 10 minutes
- Serving size: 1 omelet

NUTRITIONAL VALUES:

- Calories: 250
- Fat: 10 grams
- Protein: 15 grams
- Carbohydrates: 30 grams
- Fiber: 5 grams

INGREDIENTS:

- 1/2 cup chickpea flour
- 1/2 teaspoon baking powder
- 1/4 teaspoon turmeric
- 1/4 teaspoon salt
- 1/4 teaspoon black pepper
- 1 tablespoon water
- 1 tablespoon olive oil
- 1/4 cup chopped veggies (such as onions, peppers, mushrooms)
- 1/4 cup vegan cheese

INSTRUCTIONS:

1. In a medium bowl, mix together the chickpea flour, baking powder, turmeric, salt, and pepper.
2. Add the water and olive oil to the bowl and whisk until the batter is smooth.
3. Heat a large nonstick skillet over medium heat.
4. Pour the batter into the skillet and spread it out evenly.
5. Cook for 5 minutes, or until the omelet is cooked through and golden brown.
6. Top with the chopped veggies and vegan cheese and fold the omelet in half.
7. Serve immediately.

FLUFFY PANCAKES

- Prep time: 5 minutes
- Cooking time: 10 minutes
- Serving size: 3 pancakes

NUTRITIONAL VALUES:

- Calories: 200
- Fat: 5 grams
- Protein: 10 grams
- Carbohydrates: 30 grams
- Fiber: 4 grams

INGREDIENTS:

- 1 cup gluten-free oat flour
- 1/2 cup almond milk
- 1/4 cup unsweetened applesauce

- 1 tablespoon baking powder
- 1 teaspoon vanilla extract
- 1/2 teaspoon cinnamon
- 1/4 cup maple syrup
- 1 tablespoon olive oil
- 1/2 cup fresh or frozen berries

INSTRUCTIONS:

1. In a medium bowl, mix together the oat flour, almond milk, applesauce, baking powder, vanilla extract, and cinnamon.
2. Heat a large nonstick skillet over medium heat.
3. Pour 1/4 cup of batter into the griddle for each pancake.
4. Cook for 2-3 minutes each side, or until the pancakes are cooked through and fluffy.
5. Top with maple syrup and berries and serve immediately.

BISCUITS AND MUSHROOM GRAVY

- **Prep time: 15 minutes**
- **Cooking time: 30 minutes**
- **Serving size: 2 biscuits and 1/2 cup gravy**

NUTRITIONAL VALUES:

- Calories: 350
- Fat: 15 grams
- Protein: 10 grams
- Carbohydrates: 50 grams
- Fiber: 5 grams

INGREDIENTS:

Biscuits:

- 2 cups gluten-free all-purpose flour
- 2 teaspoons baking powder
- 1/2 teaspoon salt
- 1/4 teaspoon baking soda
- 1/4 cup vegan butter, cooled and sliced into tiny cubes
- 1 cup almond milk

Gravy:

- 1 tablespoon olive oil
- 1 onion, chopped
- 2 cloves garlic, minced
- 1 cup mushrooms, sliced
- 1/4 cup all-purpose flour
- 4 cups vegetable broth
- 1/2 teaspoon salt
- 1/4 teaspoon black pepper

INSTRUCTIONS:

Biscuits:

1. Preheat oven to 400 degrees F (200 degrees C).

2. In a large basin, mix together the flour, baking powder, salt, and baking soda.

3. Cut in the vegan butter using a pastry cutter or two knives until the mixture resembles coarse crumbs.

4. Gradually add the almond milk, mixing until the dough barely comes together.

5. Turn the dough out onto a lightly floured surface and knead gently for a few seconds.

6. Roll out the dough to 1/2-inch thickness.

7. Cut out biscuits using a 2-inch biscuit cutter.

8. Place the biscuits on a baking sheet and bake for 12-15 minutes, or until golden brown.

Gravy:

1. While the biscuits are baking, heat the olive oil in a big skillet over medium heat.

2. Add the onion and simmer until softened, approximately 5 minutes.

3. Add the garlic and mushrooms and simmer until the mushrooms are browned, approximately 5 minutes longer.

4. Sprinkle the flour over the veggies and mix to coat.

5. Cook for 1 minute, stirring regularly.

6. Gradually whisk in the veggie broth until the gravy is smooth and thick.

7. Season with salt and pepper to taste.

8. Serve the biscuits hot with the gravy.

Tips:

1. For added flavor, add 1/4 teaspoon dried thyme to the gravy.

2. If you don't have a biscuit cutter, you may use a drinking glass or a sharp knife to cut out the biscuits.

3. Leftover biscuits may be kept in an airtight jar at room temperature for up to 2 days.

OATMEAL-PECAN WAFFLES

- Prep time: 10 minutes
- Cooking time: 15 minutes
- Serving size: 2 waffles

NUTRITIONAL VALUES:

- Calories: 300
- Fat: 10 grams
- Protein: 10 grams
- Carbohydrates: 40 grams
- Fiber: 5 grams

INGREDIENTS:

- 1 cup gluten-free rolled oats
- 1/2 cup almond flour
- 2 teaspoons baking powder

- 1/2 teaspoon salt
- 1 tbsp. cinnamon
- 1/2 cup chopped pecans
- 1 1/2 cups almond milk
- 2 tablespoons maple syrup

INSTRUCTIONS:

1. Preheat waffle iron to medium heat.
2. In a blender, mix the oats, almond flour, baking powder, salt, and cinnamon.
3. Blend until the mixture is smooth.
4. Add the nuts, almond milk, and maple syrup to the blender and process until completely incorporated.
5. Pour the batter onto the waffle iron and cook until golden brown.
6. Serve immediately with your preferred toppings.

CHICKPEA FLOUR GRANOLA

- **Prep time: 10 minutes**
- **Cooking time: 20 minutes**
- **Serving size: 1/2 cup**

NUTRITIONAL VALUES:

- Calories: 200
- Fat: 10 grams
- Protein: 10 grams
- Carbohydrates: 25 grams
- Fiber: 5 grams

INGREDIENTS:

- 1 cup chickpea flour
- 1/2 cup rolled oats
- 1/4 cup chopped nuts (such as almonds, pecans, walnuts)
- 1/4 cup chia seeds
- 1/4 cup maple syrup
- 1/4 cup coconut oil, melted
- 1 teaspoon vanilla extract

INSTRUCTIONS:

1. Preheat oven to 350 degrees F (175 degrees C).
2. In a large bowl, mix the chickpea flour, oats, almonds, and chia seeds.
3. In a separate dish, mix together the maple syrup, coconut oil, and vanilla extract.
4. Pour the wet ingredients into the dry ingredients and stir until completely blended.
5. Spread the granola out onto a baking sheet and bake for 20 minutes, or until golden brown.
6. Let the granola cool fully before storing in an airtight container at room temperature.

CARROT CAKE DONUTS

- Prep time: 15 minutes
- Cooking time: 20 minutes
- Serving size: 4 donuts

NUTRITIONAL VALUES:

- Calories: 300
- Fat: 15 grams
- Protein: 5 grams
- Carbohydrates: 40 grams
- Fiber: 5 grams

INGREDIENTS:

- 1 cup gluten-free all-purpose flour
- 1 teaspoon baking powder
- 1/2 teaspoon baking soda
- 1 teaspoon cinnamon
- 1/4 teaspoon nutmeg
- 1/4 teaspoon salt
- 1 cup grated carrots
- 1/2 cup applesauce
- 1/4 cup maple syrup
- 2 tablespoons olive oil
- 1 teaspoon vanilla extract
- 1/4 cup vegan cream cheese, softened

INSTRUCTIONS:

1. Preheat oven to 350 degrees F (175 degrees C).
2. Grease a donut pans with vegan butter or frying spray.
3. In a large basin, mix together the flour, baking powder, baking soda, cinnamon, nutmeg, and salt.
4. In a second dish, mix together the carrots, applesauce, maple syrup, olive oil, and vanilla extract.
5. Add the wet ingredients to the dry ingredients and stir until just mixed.
6. Spoon the batter into the donut pan, filling each shape approximately 2/3 full.
7. Bake for 15-20 minutes, or until the donuts are golden brown and a toothpick inserted into the middle comes out clean.
8. Let the donuts cool in the pan for a few minutes before moving them to a wire rack to cool fully.

SPICED ALMOND BUTTER QUESADILLAS

- Prep time: 5 minutes
- Cooking time: 5 minutes
- Serving size: 1 quesadilla

NUTRITIONAL VALUES:

- Calories: 300
- Fat: 20 grams
- Protein: 10 grams

- Carbohydrates: 30 grams
- Fiber: 5 grams

INGREDIENTS:

- 1 tortilla, gluten-free
- 2 tbsp. almond butter
- 1/4 teaspoon ground cinnamon
- 1/8 teaspoon ground ginger
- 1/8 teaspoon ground nutmeg
- Pinch of ground cloves
- Fresh fruit, for topping (optional)

INSTRUCTIONS:

1. In a small bowl, whisk together the almond butter, cinnamon, ginger, nutmeg, and cloves.
2. Spread the almond butter mixture equally on one side of the tortilla.
3. Fold the tortilla in half, pushing down slightly to close.
4. Heat a large nonstick skillet over medium heat.
5. Place the tortilla in the pan and heat for 2-3 minutes each side, or until golden brown and the cheese has melted.
6. Cut the quesadilla into wedges and serve with fresh fruit, if preferred.

Tips:

1. For a sweeter quesadilla, add a tablespoon of maple syrup or honey to the almond butter mixture.
2. If you don't have a nonstick pan, you may use a conventional skillet gently coated with oil or vegan butter.
3. Leftover quesadillas may be kept in an airtight container at room temperature for up to 2 days.

VERY BERRY VANILLA SMOOTHIE

- **Prep time: 5 minutes**
- **Cooking time: 0 minutes**
- **Serving size: 1 smoothie**

NUTRITIONAL VALUES:

- Calories: 200
- Fat: 5 grams
- Protein: 5 grams
- Carbohydrates: 40 grams
- Fiber: 5 grams

INGREDIENTS:

- 1 cup frozen mixed berries
- 1/2 cup vanilla almond milk
- 1/2 cup plain Greek yogurt
- 1 tablespoon maple syrup
- 1/2 teaspoon vanilla extract

INSTRUCTIONS:

1. In a blender, add all of the ingredients and blend until smooth.
2. Serve immediately.

SWEET POTATO WAFFLED TOFU

- Prep time: 10 minutes
- Cooking time: 20 minutes
- Serving size: 2 waffles

NUTRITIONAL VALUES:

- Calories: 300
- Fat: 10 grams
- Protein: 15 grams
- Carbohydrates: 40 grams
- Fiber: 5 grams

INGREDIENTS:

- 1 cup mashed sweet potato
- 1/2 cup crushed tofu
- 1/4 cup chickpea flour
- 1/4 cup unsweetened applesauce
- 1 tablespoon maple syrup
- 1 teaspoon vanilla extract
- 1/2 teaspoon cinnamon
- 1/4 teaspoon nutmeg

INSTRUCTIONS:

1. Preheat waffle iron to medium heat.
2. In a large basin, mash the sweet potato.
3. Crumble the tofu and add it to the bowl.
4. Add the chickpea flour, applesauce, maple syrup, vanilla extract, cinnamon, and nutmeg to the bowl and mix thoroughly.
5. Cook the batter in the waffle iron according to the manufacturer's instructions.
6. Serve immediately with your preferred toppings.

SWEET POTATO HASH WITH ADOBO

- Prep time: 10 minutes
- Cooking time: 20 minutes
- Serving size: 2 servings

NUTRITIONAL VALUES:

- Calories: 250
- Fat: 10 grams
- Protein: 5 grams
- Carbohydrates: 35 grams
- Fiber: 5 grams

INGREDIENTS:

- 1 medium sweet potato, peeled and chopped

- 1 tablespoon olive oil
- 1/2 cup chopped onion
- 1 tablespoon adobo seasoning
- 1/4 cup chopped fresh cilantro

INSTRUCTIONS:

1. Heat the olive oil in a large pan over medium heat.
2. Add the onion and simmer until softened, approximately 5 minutes.
3. Add the sweet potato and adobo spice and simmer until the sweet potato is cooked, approximately 15 minutes.
4. Stir in the cilantro and serve immediately.

SCRAMBLED TOFU–STUFFED BREAKFAST PEPPERS

- Prep time: 15 minutes
- Cooking time: 20 minutes
- Serving size: 2 peppers

NUTRITIONAL VALUES:

- Calories: 300
- Fat: 10 grams
- Protein: 15 grams
- Carbohydrates: 40 grams
- Fiber: 5 grams

INGREDIENTS:

- 2 bell peppers, halved and seeded
- 1 block firm tofu, crumbled
- 1 tablespoon olive oil
- 1/2 cup chopped onion
- 1/2 cup chopped mushrooms
- 1/4 cup chopped spinach
- 1/4 cup chopped vegan cheese
- 1/4 teaspoon turmeric
- 1/4 teaspoon salt
- 1/4 teaspoon black pepper

INSTRUCTIONS:

1. Preheat oven to 350 degrees F (175 degrees C).
2. Heat the olive oil in a large pan over medium heat.
3. Add the onion and simmer until softened, approximately 5 minutes.
4. Add the mushrooms and sauté until browned, approximately 5 minutes longer.
5. Add the spinach and heat until wilted, approximately 1 minute.
6. Stir in the tofu, turmeric, salt, and pepper.
7. Spoon the tofu mixture into the pepper halves.
8. Sprinkle the vegan cheese over the top.
9. Bake for 15-20 minutes, or until the peppers are soft.

STRAWBERRY BREAKFAST BRUSCHETTA

- Prep time: 5 minutes
- Cooking time: 0 minutes
- Serving size: 2 servings

NUTRITIONAL VALUES:

- Calories: 200
- Fat: 5 grams
- Protein: 5 grams
- Carbohydrates: 35 grams
- Fiber: 4 grams

INGREDIENTS:

- 2 slices crusty gluten-free bread
- 1/2 cup sliced strawberries
- 1/4 cup chopped fresh basil
- 1 tablespoon balsamic vinegar
- 1 tablespoon olive oil
- Salt and pepper to taste

INSTRUCTIONS:

1. Toast the bread till just golden brown.
2. In a small bowl, mix the strawberries, basil, balsamic vinegar, and olive oil.
3. Season with salt and pepper to taste.
4. Spread the strawberry mixture on the bread.
5. Serve immediately.

JICAMA HASH BROWNS

- Prep time: 10 minutes
- Cooking time: 20 minutes
- Serving size: 2 servings

NUTRITIONAL VALUES:

- Calories: 200
- Fat: 10 grams
- Protein: 5 grams
- Carbohydrates: 25 grams
- Fiber: 5 grams

INGREDIENTS:

- 1 medium jicama, peeled and grated
- 1 tablespoon olive oil
- 1/2 cup chopped onion
- 1/4 cup sliced bell pepper
- 1/4 teaspoon salt
- 1/4 teaspoon black pepper

INSTRUCTIONS:

1. Heat the olive oil in a large pan over medium heat.
2. Add the onion and simmer until softened, approximately 5 minutes.
3. Add the jicama and bell pepper and simmer until the jicama is soft, approximately 15 minutes.
4. Season with salt and pepper to taste.
5. Serve immediately.

CINNAMON ROLLS

- Prep time: 20 minutes
- Cooking time: 30 minutes
- Serving size: 4 rolls

NUTRITIONAL VALUES:

- Calories: 300
- Fat: 15 grams
- Protein: 5 grams
- Carbohydrates: 40 grams
- Fiber: 5 grams

INGREDIENTS:

Dough:

- 1 cup gluten-free all-purpose flour
- 1 tablespoon baking powder
- 1/2 teaspoon salt
- 1/4 cup vegan butter, softened
- 1/2 cup unsweetened applesauce
- 1/4 cup almond milk

Filling:

- 1/4 cup vegan butter, softened
- 1/4 cup packed light brown sugar
- 1 tablespoon ground cinnamon

Icing:

- 1/2 cup powdered sugar
- 1 tablespoon almond milk
- 1/2 teaspoon vanilla extract

INSTRUCTIONS:

Dough:

1. In a large bowl, mix together the flour, baking powder, and salt.
2. Cut in the vegan butter using a pastry cutter or two knives until the mixture resembles coarse crumbs.
3. Gradually add the applesauce and almond milk, mixing until the dough barely comes together.
4. Turn the dough out onto a lightly floured surface and knead gently for a few seconds.
5. Roll out the dough into a 12x16 inch rectangle.

Filling:

1. In a small bowl, mix together the vegan butter, brown sugar, and cinnamon until smooth.
2. Spread the contents evenly over the dough.
3. Roll up the dough from the long end, jelly-roll style.
4. Cut the roll into 12 pieces.
5. Place the rolls in a greased 9x13 inch baking dish.

6. Bake at 350 degrees F (175 degrees C) for 25-30 minutes, or until golden brown.

Icing:

1. In a small bowl, mix together the powdered sugar, almond milk, and vanilla extract until smooth.
2. Drizzle the frosting over the cinnamon rolls.
3. Serve immediately.

TRIPLE BERRY TOASTY TARTS

- **Prep time: 10 minutes**
- **Cooking time: 20 minutes**
- **Serving size: 4 tarts**

NUTRITIONAL VALUES:

- Calories: 250
- Fat: 10 grams
- Protein: 5 grams
- Carbohydrates: 35 grams
- Fiber: 5 grams

INGREDIENTS:

- 4 slices gluten-free bread
- 1/4 cup mixed berries (such as strawberries, blueberries, raspberries)
- 1 tablespoon cornstarch
- 1 tablespoon maple syrup
- 1/4 teaspoon vanilla extract
- 1 tablespoon vegan butter, softened
- 1/4 cup powdered sugar
- 1 tablespoon almond milk

INSTRUCTIONS:

1. Preheat oven to 400 degrees F (200 degrees C).
2. In a small dish, mix the berries, cornstarch, maple syrup, and vanilla extract.
3. Place 1/4 cup of the berry mixture in the middle of each piece of bread.
4. Fold the bread into a square, pressing the edges to seal.
5. Melt the vegan butter in a large pan over medium heat.
6. Place the bread squares in the pan and heat until golden brown on both sides, approximately 3 minutes each side.
7. In a small bowl, mix together the powdered sugar and almond milk until smooth.
8. Drizzle the frosting over the toasted tarts.
9. Serve immediately.

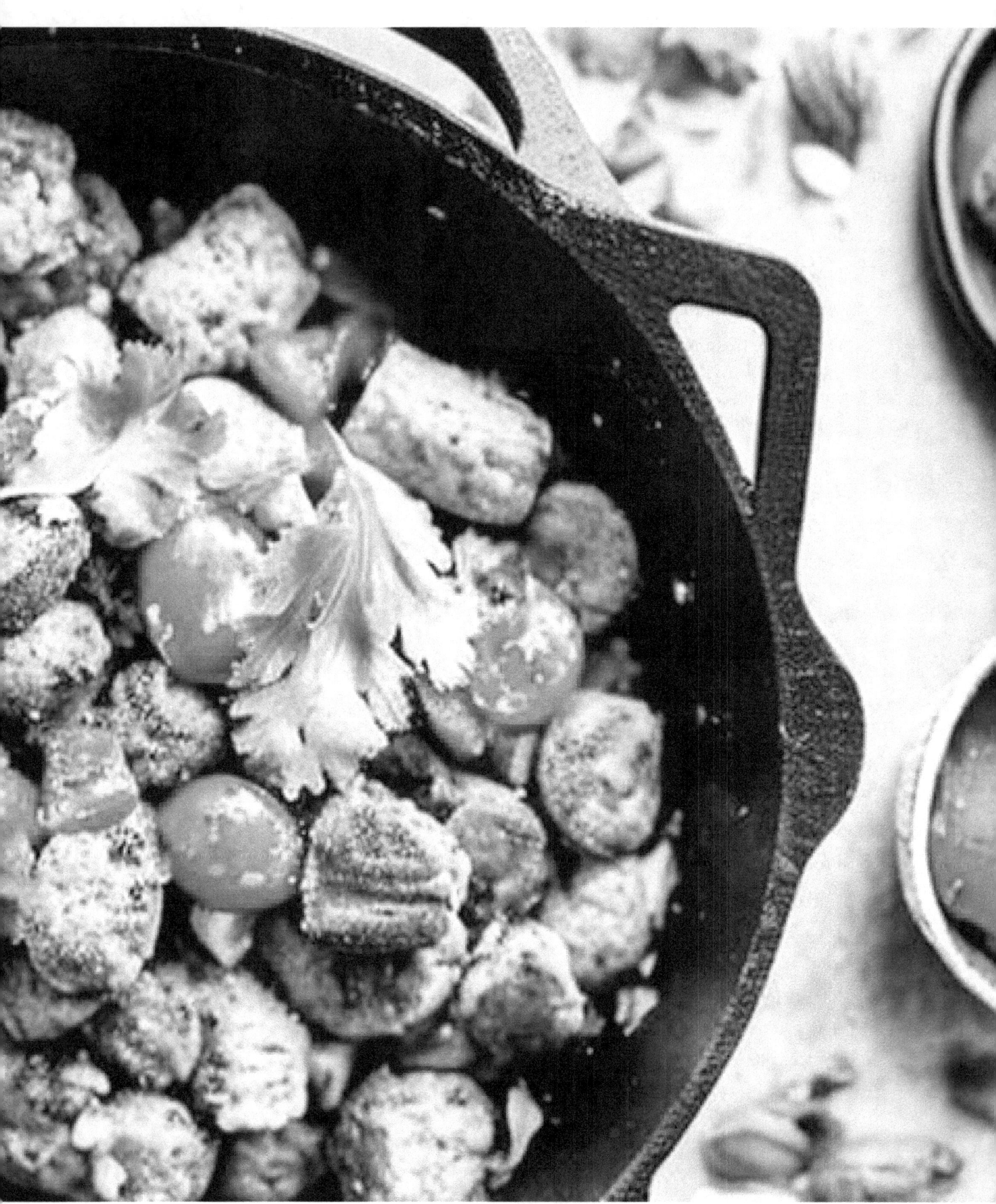

PEACH AND BASIL CAPRESE SALAD

- Prep time: 5 minutes
- Cooking time: 0 minutes
- Serving size: 2 servings

NUTRITIONAL VALUES:

- Calories: 200
- Fat: 10 grams
- Protein: 5 grams
- Carbohydrates: 25 grams
- Fiber: 5 grams

INGREDIENTS:

- 2 cups sliced peaches
- 1/2 cup chopped fresh basil
- 1/4 cup balsamic vinegar
- 1 tablespoon olive oil
- Salt and pepper to taste

INSTRUCTIONS:

1. Combine the peaches, basil, balsamic vinegar, olive oil, salt, and pepper in a large bowl.
2. Toss to coat.
3. Serve immediately.

WEDGE SALAD WITH GLUTEN-FREE CROUTONS

- Prep time: 10 minutes
- Cooking time: 10 minutes
- Serving size: 2 servings

NUTRITIONAL VALUES:

- Calories: 300
- Fat: 15 grams
- Protein: 5 grams
- Carbohydrates: 35 grams
- Fiber: 5 grams

INGREDIENTS:

- 1 head iceberg lettuce, cut into wedges
- 1/2 cup sliced cherry tomatoes
- 1/4 cup chopped red onion
- 1/4 cup gluten-free croutons
- 1/4 cup balsamic vinaigrette

INSTRUCTIONS:

1. Preheat oven to 350 degrees F (175 degrees C).
2. Cut the bread into 1-inch pieces.
3. Drizzle the bread cubes with olive oil and season with salt and pepper.

4. Spread the bread cubes on a baking sheet and bake for 10 minutes, or until golden brown.

5. In a large bowl, mix the lettuce, tomatoes, red onion, and croutons.

6. Drizzle with balsamic vinaigrette and toss to coat.

7. Serve immediately.

SUNFLOWER SEED "TUNA" SANDWICHES

- Prep time: 15 minutes
- Cooking time: 0 minutes
- Serving size: 2 sandwiches

NUTRITIONAL VALUES:

- Calories: 300
- Fat: 15 grams
- Protein: 10 grams
- Carbohydrates: 30 grams
- Fiber: 5 grams

INGREDIENTS:

- 1/2 cup sunflower seeds
- 1/4 cup chopped celery
- 1/4 cup chopped red onion
- 1/4 cup vegan mayonnaise
- 1 tablespoon lemon juice
- 1/2 teaspoon salt
- 1/4 teaspoon black pepper
- 2 slices gluten-free bread

INSTRUCTIONS:

1. In a food processor, pulse the sunflower seeds until they resemble breadcrumbs.

2. In a large bowl, mix the sunflower seed crumbs, celery, red onion, vegan mayonnaise, lemon juice, salt, and pepper.

3. Spread the sunflower seed mixture on the bread.

4. Serve immediately.

CHICKPEA CAESAR SALAD WRAP

- Prep time: 10 minutes
- Cooking time: 0 minutes
- Serving size: 2 wraps

NUTRITIONAL VALUES:

- Calories: 300
- Fat: 10 grams
- Protein: 15 grams
- Carbohydrates: 40 grams
- Fiber: 5 grams

INGREDIENTS:

- 1 cup cooked chickpeas, mashed
- 1/4 cup vegan Caesar dressing

- 1/4 cup chopped romaine lettuce
- 1/4 cup chopped cherry tomatoes
- 2 gluten-free tortillas

INSTRUCTIONS:

1. In a large bowl, mix the mashed chickpeas, vegan Caesar dressing, romaine lettuce, and cherry tomatoes.
2. Spread the chickpea Caesar salad mixture equally on the tortillas.
3. Roll up the tortillas and serve immediately.

CRISPY HEARTS OF PALM PO' BOY

- **Prep time: 15 minutes**
- **Cooking time: 20 minutes**
- **Serving size: 2 sandwiches**

NUTRITIONAL VALUES:

- Calories: 350
- Fat: 20 grams
- Protein: 10 grams
- Carbohydrates: 40 grams
- Fiber: 5 grams

INGREDIENTS:

- 1 can (15 ounces) hearts of palm, drained and sliced
- 1/2 cup gluten-free bread crumbs
- 1/4 cup cornstarch
- 1 teaspoon paprika
- 1/2 teaspoon salt
- 1/4 teaspoon black pepper
- 1/4 cup vegan mayonnaise
- 2 tbsp. vegan sriracha
- 2 gluten-free hoagie rolls

INSTRUCTIONS:

In a large bowl, mix the bread crumbs, cornstarch, paprika, salt, and pepper.

1. Dredge the hearts of palm slices in the bread crumb mixture.
2. Heat a large skillet over medium heat.
3. Add 1/4 cup of vegetable oil to the skillet.
4. Fry the hearts of palm slices in batches until golden brown and crispy, approximately 2-3 minutes each batch.
5. In a small bowl, mix the vegan mayonnaise and vegan sriracha.
6. Spread the sriracha mayonnaise on the bottom buns of the hoagie rolls.
7. Top with the crispy hearts of palm slices.
8. Close the sandwiches and serve immediately.

1. For extra crispy hearts of palm, you may double-dredge them in the bread crumb mixture.
2. If you don't have vegan sriracha, you may substitute any other spicy sauce that you prefer.
3. You may also use different varieties of bread; such as gluten-free baguettes or ciabatta rolls.

EGGPLANT BACON "E-L-T"

- **Prep time: 20 minutes**
- **Cooking time: 20 minutes**
- **Serving size: 2 sandwiches**

NUTRITIONAL VALUES:

- Calories: 300
- Fat: 15 grams
- Protein: 10 grams
- Carbohydrates: 35 grams
- Fiber: 5 grams

INGREDIENTS:

- 1 medium eggplant, cut
- 1 tablespoon olive oil
- 1 tablespoon soy sauce
- 1 teaspoon liquid smoke
- 1/4 teaspoon smoked paprika
- 1/4 teaspoon salt
- 1/4 teaspoon black pepper
- 2 slices gluten-free bread
- 1/2 cup lettuce
- 1 tomato, sliced

INSTRUCTIONS:

1. Preheat oven to 400 degrees F (200 degrees C).
2. In a medium bowl, mix the olive oil, soy sauce, liquid smoke, smoked paprika, salt, and pepper.
3. Add the eggplant slices to the bowl and toss to coat.
4. Spread the eggplant slices in a single layer on a baking sheet.
5. Bake for 20 minutes, or until the eggplant is soft and golden.
6. To prepare the sandwiches, put the eggplant slices on the bread.
7. Top with lettuce and tomato.
8. Serve immediately.

COCONUT CORN CHOWDER

- **Prep time: 15 minutes**
- **Cooking time: 30 minutes**
- **Serving size: 4 servings**

NUTRITIONAL VALUES:

- Calories: 250
- Fat: 15 grams
- Protein: 5 grams

- Carbohydrates: 30 grams
- Fiber: 5 grams

INGREDIENTS:

- 1 tablespoon olive oil
- 1 onion, chopped
- 2 cloves garlic, minced
- 4 cups vegetable broth
- 1 cup frozen corn
- 1 cup coconut milk
- 1/2 cup chopped tomatoes
- 1/4 cup chopped cilantro
- Salt and pepper to taste

INSTRUCTIONS:

1. Heat the olive oil in a big saucepan over medium heat.
2. Add the onion and simmer until softened, approximately 5 minutes.
3. Add the garlic and simmer for 1 minute longer.
4. Add the vegetable broth, corn, coconut milk, tomatoes, and cilantro.
5. Bring to a boil, then decrease heat and simmer for 20 minutes.
6. Season with salt and pepper to taste.
7. Serve hot.

SAMOSA WRAP

- **Prep time: 10 minutes**
- **Cooking time: 15 minutes**
- **Serving size: 2 wraps**

NUTRITIONAL VALUES:

- Calories: 300
- Fat: 15 grams
- Protein: 10 grams
- Carbohydrates: 35 grams
- Fiber: 5 grams

INGREDIENTS:

- 1 cup cooked chickpeas, mashed
- 1/2 cup chopped red onion
- 1/4 cup chopped cilantro
- 1 tablespoon curry powder
- 1 teaspoon turmeric
- 1/2 teaspoon salt
- 1/4 teaspoon black pepper
- 2 gluten-free tortillas

INSTRUCTIONS:

1. In a large bowl, mix the mashed chickpeas, red onion, cilantro, curry powder, turmeric, salt, and pepper.
2. Spread the samosa contents equally on the tortillas.
3. Roll up the tortillas and serve immediately.

BALSAMIC MUSHROOM AND QUINOA LETTUCE WRAPS

- Prep time: 15 minutes
- Cooking time: 20 minutes
- Serving size: 4 wraps

NUTRITIONAL VALUES:

- Calories: 350
- Fat: 15 grams
- Protein: 10 grams
- Carbohydrates: 40 grams
- Fiber: 5 grams

INGREDIENTS:

- 1 tablespoon olive oil
- 1 onion, chopped
- 2 cloves garlic, minced
- 8 ounces mushrooms, sliced
- 1/4 cup balsamic vinegar
- 1/4 cup cooked quinoa
- 1/4 cup chopped fresh basil
- Salt and pepper to taste
- 4 lettuce leaves

INSTRUCTIONS:

1. Heat the olive oil in a large pan over medium heat.
2. Add the onion and simmer until softened, approximately 5 minutes.
3. Add the garlic and simmer for 1 minute longer.
4. Add the mushrooms and sauté until browned, approximately 5 minutes longer.
5. Stir in the balsamic vinegar, quinoa, and basil.
6. Season with salt and pepper to taste

SIMPLE TOMATO SOUP

- Prep time: 10 minutes
- Cooking time: 20 minutes
- Serving size: 4 servings

NUTRITIONAL VALUES:

- Calories: 150
- Fat: 5 grams
- Protein: 5 grams
- Carbohydrates: 25 grams
- Fiber: 5 grams

INGREDIENTS:

- 1 tablespoon olive oil
- 1 onion, chopped
- 2 cloves garlic, minced
- 28 ounces mashed tomatoes
- 1 tablespoon dried oregano
- 1/2 teaspoon salt
- 1/4 teaspoon black pepper

INSTRUCTIONS:

1. Heat the olive oil in a big saucepan over medium heat.

2. Add the onion and simmer until softened, approximately 5 minutes.

3. Add the garlic and simmer for 1 minute longer.

4. Add the smashed tomatoes, oregano, salt, and pepper.

5. Bring to a boil, then decrease heat and simmer for 15 minutes.

6. Serve hot.

ROOT VEGETABLE AND SORGHUM STEW

- Prep time: 20 minutes
- Cooking time: 40 minutes
- Serving size: 4 servings

NUTRITIONAL VALUES:

- Calories: 300
- Fat: 10 grams
- Protein: 10 grams
- Carbohydrates: 40 grams
- Fiber: 10 grams

INGREDIENTS:

- 1 tablespoon olive oil
- 1 onion, chopped
- 2 carrots, chopped
- 2 celery stalks, chopped
- 1 parsnip, chopped
- 1 cup sorghum, washed
- 4 cups vegetable broth
- 1 teaspoon dried thyme
- 1/2 teaspoon salt
- 1/4 teaspoon black pepper

INSTRUCTIONS:

1. Heat the olive oil in a big saucepan over medium heat.

2. Add the onion and simmer until softened, approximately 5 minutes.

3. Add the carrots, celery, and parsnip and simmer for 5 minutes longer.

4. Add the sorghum, vegetable broth, thyme, salt, and pepper.

5. Bring to a boil, then decrease heat and simmer for 30 minutes, or until the sorghum is soft.

6. Serve hot.

BORSCHT

- Prep time: 15 minutes
- Cooking time: 45 minutes
- Serving size: 4 servings

NUTRITIONAL VALUES:

- Calories: 250
- Fat: 5 grams
- Protein: 10 grams
- Carbohydrates: 40 grams

Fiber: 5 grams

INGREDIENTS:

- 1 tablespoon olive oil
- 1 onion, chopped
- 2 cloves garlic, minced
- 1 beet, chopped
- 2 carrots, chopped
- 2 cups vegetable broth
- 1 cup shredded cabbage
- 1/2 cup canned diced tomatoes
- 1 tablespoon tomato paste
- 1 teaspoon dried dill
- 1/2 teaspoon salt
- 1/4 teaspoon black pepper

INSTRUCTIONS:

1. Heat the olive oil in a big saucepan over medium heat.
2. Add the onion and simmer until softened, approximately 5 minutes.
3. Add the garlic, beet, and carrots and simmer for 5 minutes longer.
4. Add the vegetable broth, cabbage, diced tomatoes, tomato paste, dill, salt, and pepper.
5. Bring to a boil, then decrease heat and simmer for 30 minutes, or until the veggies are soft.
6. Serve hot.

CREAMY ZUPPA TOSCANA

- Prep time: 15 minutes
- Cooking time: 30 minutes
- Serving size: 4 servings

NUTRITIONAL VALUES:

- Calories: 300
- Fat: 15 grams
- Protein: 10 grams
- Carbohydrates: 35 grams
- Fiber: 5 grams

INGREDIENTS:

- 1 tablespoon olive oil
- 1 onion, chopped
- 2 cloves garlic, minced
- 4 cups vegetable broth
- 1 pound Italian sausage, removed from casings
- 4 russet potatoes, peeled and diced
- 1/2 cup chopped kale
- 1 1/2 cups heavy cream
- Salt and pepper to taste
- Crushed red pepper flakes to taste, if desired

INSTRUCTIONS:

1. Heat the olive oil in a big saucepan over medium heat.

2. Add the onion and simmer until softened, approximately 5 minutes.

3. Add the garlic and simmer for 1 minute longer.

4. Add the Italian sausage and heat until browned, breaking it up into tiny pieces.

5. Add the potatoes and veggie broth.

6. Bring to a boil, then decrease heat and simmer for 20 minutes, or until the potatoes are cooked.

7. Stir in the kale and simmer for 2 minutes, or until wilted.

8. Stir in the heavy cream and season with salt and pepper to taste.

9. Serve hot with a sprinkling of crushed red pepper flakes, if preferred.

Tips:

1. For a fuller taste, use whole milk instead of heavy cream.

2. If you don't have kale, you can use spinach instead.

3. Add a sprinkle of nutmeg to the soup for a warm and cozy taste.

CHICKPEA "CHICKEN" SOUP

- Prep time: 15 minutes
- Cooking time: 30 minutes
- Serving size: 4 servings

NUTRITIONAL VALUES:

- Calories: 300
- Fat: 10 grams
- Protein: 15 grams
- Carbohydrates: 35 grams
- Fiber: 5 grams

INGREDIENTS:

- 1 tablespoon olive oil
- 1 onion, chopped
- 2 cloves garlic, minced
- 2 carrots, chopped
- 2 celery stalks, chopped
- 1 cup dry chickpeas, soaked overnight and drained
- 4 cups vegetable broth
- 1 teaspoon dried thyme
- 1/2 teaspoon salt
- 1/4 teaspoon black pepper

INSTRUCTIONS:

1. Heat the olive oil in a big saucepan over medium heat.

2. Add the onion and simmer until softened, approximately 5 minutes.

3. Add the garlic, carrots, and celery and simmer for 5 minutes longer.

4. Add the chickpeas, vegetable broth, thyme, salt, and pepper.

5. Bring to a boil, then decrease heat and simmer for 30 minutes, or until the chickpeas are cooked.

6. Serve hot.

ROASTED BUTTERNUT SQUASH SOUP

- **Prep time: 20 minutes**
- **Cooking time: 40 minutes**
- **Serving size: 4 servings**

NUTRITIONAL VALUES:

- Calories: 250
- Fat: 10 grams
- Protein: 5 grams
- Carbohydrates: 35 grams
- Fiber: 5 grams

INGREDIENTS:

- 1 butternut squash, peeled and cubed
- 1 tablespoon olive oil
- 1 onion, chopped
- 2 cloves garlic, minced
- 4 cups vegetable broth
- 1 teaspoon ground cumin
- 1/2 teaspoon salt
- 1/4 teaspoon black pepper
- 1/4 cup chopped fresh cilantro

INSTRUCTIONS:

1. Preheat oven to 400 degrees F (200 degrees C).

2. Toss the butternut squash with olive oil, salt, and pepper.

3. Spread the butternut squash in a single layer on a baking sheet.

4. Roast for 30 minutes, or until the squash is soft.

5. Heat the olive oil in a big saucepan over medium heat.

6. Add the onion and simmer until softened, approximately 5 minutes.

7. Add the garlic and simmer for 1 minute longer.

8. Add the roasted butternut squash, vegetable broth, cumin, salt, and pepper.

9. Bring to a boil, then decrease heat and simmer for 15 minutes, or until the soup is smooth.

10. Stir in the cilantro and serve hot.

CARIBBEAN-INSPIRED SWEET POTATO SOUP

- **Prep time: 15 minutes**
- **Cooking time: 30 minutes**
- **Serving size: 4 servings**

NUTRITIONAL VALUES:

- Calories: 200
- Fat: 10 grams

- Protein: 5 grams
- Carbohydrates: 30 grams
- Fiber: 5 grams

INGREDIENTS:

- 1 tablespoon olive oil
- 1 onion, chopped
- 2 cloves garlic, minced
- 1 sweet potato, peeled and sliced
- 2 cups vegetable broth
- 1 cup canned chopped tomatoes
- 1 tablespoon coconut milk
- 1 teaspoon ground ginger
- 1/2 teaspoon salt
- 1/4 teaspoon black pepper

INSTRUCTIONS:

1. Heat the olive oil in a big saucepan over medium heat.
2. Add the onion and simmer until softened, approximately 5 minutes.
3. Add the garlic, sweet potato, and vegetable broth.
4. Bring to a boil, then decrease heat and simmer for 15 minutes, or until the sweet potato is cooked.
5. Stir in the chopped tomatoes, coconut milk, ginger, salt, and pepper.
6. Serve hot.

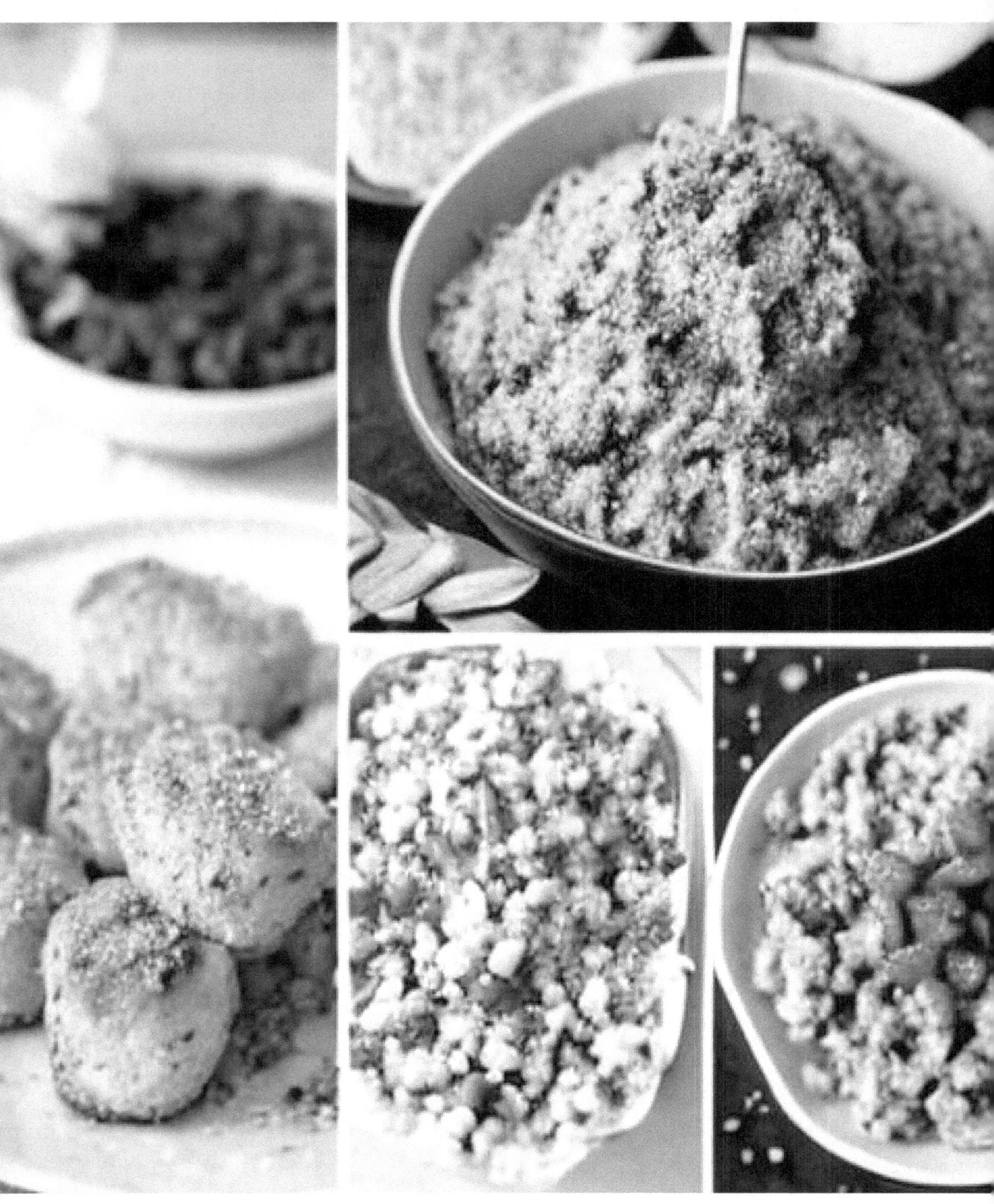

SWEET CORN PUDDING

- Prep time: 10 minutes
- Cooking time: 30 minutes
- Serving size: 4 servings

NUTRITIONAL VALUES:

- Calories: 200
- Fat: 5 grams
- Protein: 5 grams
- Carbohydrates: 35 grams
- Fiber: 5 grams

INGREDIENTS:

- 2 cups fresh corn kernels
- 1/2 cup unsweetened almond milk
- 1/4 cup gluten-free all-purpose flour
- 2 eggs
- 1 teaspoon baking powder
- 1/2 teaspoon salt
- 1/4 teaspoon black pepper

INSTRUCTIONS:

1. Preheat oven to 350 degrees F (175 degrees C).
2. Grease a 1-quart baking dish with butter.
3. In a large basin, mix the corn kernels, almond milk, flour, eggs, baking powder, salt, and pepper.
4. Pour the batter into the prepared baking dish.
5. Bake for 30 minutes, or until the pudding is set.

BRUSSELS SPROUT SLAW

- Prep time: 15 minutes
- Cooking time: 10 minutes
- Serving size: 4 servings

NUTRITIONAL VALUES:

- Calories: 150
- Fat: 10 grams
- Protein: 5 grams
- Carbohydrates: 15 grams
- Fiber: 5 grams

INGREDIENTS:

- 2 tablespoons olive oil
- 1/2 cup chopped onion 1/2 cup chopped red bell pepper
- 3 cups shredded Brussels sprouts
- 1/4 cup chopped fresh parsley
- 1/4 cup lemon juice
- 1 tablespoon Dijon mustard
- 1 teaspoon maple syrup

- Salt and pepper to taste

INSTRUCTIONS:

1. In a large bowl, mix together the olive oil, onion, and red bell pepper.
2. Add the shredded Brussels sprouts, parsley, lemon juice, Dijon mustard, maple syrup, salt, and pepper.
3. Toss to coat.
4. Serve immediately.

PINEAPPLE-CAULIFLOWER RICE

- **Prep time: 10 minutes**
- **Cooking time: 15 minutes**
- **Serving size: 4 servings**

NUTRITIONAL VALUES:

- Calories: 150
- Fat: 5 grams
- Protein: 5 grams
- Carbohydrates: 25 grams
- Fiber: 5 grams

INGREDIENTS:

- 1 head cauliflower, riced
- 1 tablespoon olive oil
- 1 onion, chopped 1 clove garlic, minced 1 cup canned pineapple pieces, drained

- 1/4 cup chopped fresh cilantro
- 1/4 cup soy sauce
- 1 tablespoon lime juice
- Salt and pepper to taste

INSTRUCTIONS:

1. Heat the olive oil in a large pan over medium heat.
2. Add the onion and simmer until softened, approximately 5 minutes.
3. Add the garlic and simmer for 1 minute longer.
4. Add the rice cauliflower and simmer for 5 minutes, or until soft.
5. Stir in the pineapple pieces, cilantro, soy sauce, lime juice, salt, and pepper.
6. Serve hot or cold.

MEDITERRANEAN PASTA SALAD

- **Prep time: 15 minutes**
- **Cooking time: 10 minutes**
- **Serving size: 4 servings**

NUTRITIONAL VALUES:

- Calories: 300
- Fat: 15 grams
- Protein: 10 grams
- Carbohydrates: 35 grams
- Fiber: 5 grams

INGREDIENTS:

- 1-pound gluten-free spaghetti
- 1/2 cup chopped cucumber
- 1/2 cup chopped cherry tomatoes
- 1/2 cup chopped red onion 1/4 cup chopped Kalamata olives
- 1/4 cup chopped fresh parsley
- 1/4 cup olive oil
- 2 teaspoons lemon juice
- 1 tablespoon dried oregano
- 1 teaspoon salt
- 1/2 teaspoon black pepper

INSTRUCTIONS:

1. Cook the pasta according per package guidelines.
2. Drain and rinse the pasta under cold water.
3. In a large bowl, add the spaghetti, cucumber, cherry tomatoes, red onion, Kalamata olives, and parsley.
4. In a small bowl, mix together the olive oil, lemon juice, oregano, salt, and pepper profile image
5. Pour the dressing over the pasta salad and toss to coat.
6. Serve immediately or refrigerate for later.

1. For a more delicious pasta salad, marinate the veggies in the dressing for 30 minutes before adding the pasta.
2. You may also add additional veggies to this pasta salad, such as sliced bell peppers, zucchini, or artichoke hearts.
3. If you don't have Kalamata olives, you may substitute any other sort of olive that you want.

CHEESY DILL CARROTS

- **Prep time: 10 minutes**
- **Cooking time: 20 minutes**
- **Serving size: 4 servings**

NUTRITIONAL VALUES:

- Calories: 150
- Fat: 10 grams
- Protein: 5 grams
- Carbohydrates: 20 grams
- Fiber: 5 grams

INGREDIENTS:

- 2 pounds' carrots, peeled and sliced
- 2 tablespoons olive oil
- 1/4 cup minced fresh dill 1/4 cup grated Parmesan cheese 1/4 teaspoon salt
- 1/4 teaspoon black pepper

INSTRUCTIONS:

INSTRUCTIONS:

1. Preheat oven to 400 degrees F (200 degrees C).
2. Toss the carrots with olive oil, dill, Parmesan cheese, salt, and pepper.
3. Spread the carrots in a single layer on a baking pan.
4. Roast for 20 minutes, or until the carrots are soft.
5. Serve hot.

MASHED CAULIFLOWER AND RUTABAGA WITH ROASTED GARLIC

- Prep time: 20 minutes
- Cooking time: 45 minutes
- Serving size: 4 servings

NUTRITIONAL VALUES:

- Calories: 200
- Fat: 5 grams
- Protein: 5 grams
- Carbohydrates: 35 grams
- Fiber: 5 grams

INGREDIENTS:

- 1 head cauliflower, cut into florets
- 1 rutabaga, peeled and cubed
- 1 head garlic, cloves separated and peeled
- 1/4 cup olive oil
- 1/4 cup unsweetened almond milk
- Salt and pepper to taste

INSTRUCTIONS:

1. Preheat oven to 400 degrees F (200 degrees C).
2. Toss the cauliflower and rutabaga with olive oil and salt.
3. Spread the veggies in a single layer on a baking sheet.
4. Roast for 20 minutes.
5. Add the garlic cloves to the baking sheet and roast for 20 minutes longer, or until the veggies are cooked and the garlic is soft.
6. In a large saucepan, mash the cauliflower, rutabaga, and garlic cloves.
7. Stir in the almond milk, salt, and pepper to taste.
8. Serve hot.

"PARMESAN" ROASTED PARSNIP FRIES

- Prep time: 15 minutes
- Cooking time: 30 minutes
- Serving size: 4 servings

NUTRITIONAL VALUES:

- Calories: 200
- Fat: 10 grams
- Protein: 5 grams
- Carbohydrates: 30 grams
- Fiber: 5 grams

INGREDIENTS:

- 2 pounds' parsnips, peeled and cut into fry
- 2 tablespoons olive oil
- 1/4 cup nutritional yeast
- 2 tablespoons cornstarch
- 1 teaspoon dried garlic powder
- 1/2 teaspoon salt
- 1/4 teaspoon black pepper

INSTRUCTIONS:

1. Preheat oven to 400 degrees F (200 degrees C).
2. Toss the parsnip fries with olive oil, nutritional yeast, cornstarch, garlic powder, salt, and pepper.
3. Spread the parsnip fries in a single layer on a baking sheet.
4. Roast for 30 minutes, or until the fries are golden brown and crispy.
5. Serve hot with your favorite dipping sauce.

BAKED MISO SWEET POTATOES

- Prep time: 10 minutes
- Cooking time: 45 minutes
- Serving size: 4 servings

NUTRITIONAL VALUES:

- Calories: 250
- Fat: 15 grams
- Protein: 5 grams
- Carbohydrates: 35 grams
- Fiber: 5 grams

INGREDIENTS:

- 4 medium sweet potatoes, pricked with a fork
- 2 tablespoons olive oil 2 teaspoons white miso paste
- 2 tablespoons maple syrup
- 1 tablespoon rice vinegar
- 1 teaspoon sesame oil
- 1/2 teaspoon minced fresh ginger
- Salt and pepper to taste

INSTRUCTIONS:

1. Preheat oven to 400 degrees F (200 degrees C).
2. In a small bowl, mix together the olive oil, miso paste, maple syrup, rice

vinegar, sesame oil, ginger, salt, and
pepper.

3. Brush the miso mixture over the sweet
potatoes.

4. Place the sweet potatoes on a baking
sheet and bake for 45 minutes, or until
soft and caramelized profile picture

GARLIC BUTTER RICE WITH KALE AND MUSHROOMS

- Prep Time: 20 minutes
- Cook Time: 20 minutes
- Serving Size: 4 servings

INGREDIENTS:

- 1 cup gluten-free rice
- 1 tablespoon olive oil
- 1/2 onion, chopped
- 2 cloves garlic, minced
- 1 cup sliced mushrooms
- 1 cup chopped kale
- 1/4 cup vegan butter
- Salt and pepper to taste

INSTRUCTIONS:

1. Cook the rice according per package
guidelines.

2. While the rice is cooking, heat the
olive oil in a large pan over medium
heat.

3. Add the onion and simmer until
softened, approximately 5 minutes.

4. Add the garlic and simmer for 1
minute longer.

5. Add the mushrooms and sauté until
browned, approximately 5 minutes
longer.

6. Add the greens and simmer until
wilted, approximately 2 minutes.

7. Stir in the vegan butter and season with
salt & pepper to taste.

8. Serve over the prepared rice.

PUMPKIN AND SAGE RISOTTO

- Prep Time: 15 minutes
- Cook Time: 30 minutes
- Serving Size: 4 servings

INGREDIENTS:

- 1 tablespoon olive oil
- 1 onion, chopped
- 2 cloves garlic, minced
- 1 cup canned pumpkin puree
- 1/2 cup gluten-free vegetable broth 1/4
cup chopped fresh sage
- 1/4 cup vegan Parmesan cheese
- Salt and pepper to taste

INSTRUCTIONS:

1. Heat the olive oil in a big saucepan over medium heat.
2. Add the onion and simmer until softened, approximately 5 minutes.
3. Add the garlic and simmer for 1 minute longer.
4. Add the pumpkin puree, vegetable broth, sage, and vegan Parmesan cheese.
5. Bring to a boil, then decrease heat and simmer for 20 minutes, or until the risotto is thick and creamy.
6. Season with salt and pepper to taste.
7. Serve hot.

AMARANTH AND WALNUT PILAF

- Prep Time: 10 minutes
- Cook Time: 20 minutes
- Serving Size: 4 servings

INGREDIENTS:

- 1 cup amaranth grain
- 1 tablespoon olive oil
- 1 onion, chopped
- 2 cloves garlic, minced
- 1 cup chopped walnuts
- 1/2 cup chopped fresh parsley
- 1/4 cup vegetable broth
- Salt and pepper to taste

INSTRUCTIONS:

1. Rinse the amaranth grain in a fine mesh sieve.
2. Heat the olive oil in a big saucepan over medium heat.
3. Add the onion and simmer until softened, approximately 5 minutes.
4. Add the garlic and simmer for 1 minute longer.
5. Add the amaranth, walnuts, parsley, and vegetable broth.
6. Bring to a boil, then decrease heat and simmer for 15 minutes, or until the amaranth is cooked through and the liquid is absorbed.
7. Season with salt and pepper to taste.
8. Serve hot.

HASSELBACK POTATOES

- Prep Time: 20 minutes
- Cook Time: 1 hour
- Serving Size: 4 servings

INGREDIENTS:

- 4 big russet potatoes
- 2 tablespoons olive oil
- Salt and pepper to taste

INSTRUCTIONS:

1. Preheat oven to 400 degrees F (200 degrees C).
2. Wash the potatoes and pat them dry.
3. Place the potatoes on a chopping board and gently slice them thinly, leaving them connected at the bottom.
4. In a small bowl, add the olive oil, salt, and pepper.
5. Brush the oil mixture over the potatoes.
6. Place the potatoes on a baking sheet and roast for 1 hour, or until the potatoes are soft and cooked through.
7. Serve hot.

ROASTED CARROTS WITH FENNEL

- Prep Time: 15 minutes
- Cook Time: 30 minutes
- Serving Size: 4 servings

INGREDIENTS:

- 1 pound carrots, peeled and cut into bits
- 1 bulb fennel, trimmed and sliced into bits
- 2 tablespoons olive oil
- Salt and pepper to taste

INSTRUCTIONS:

- Preheat oven to 400 degrees F (200 degrees C).
- Toss the carrots and fennel with olive oil, salt, and pepper.
- Spread the veggies in a single layer on a baking sheet.
- Roast for 30 minutes, or until the veggies are soft and slightly browned.

WILD RICE WITH BROCCOLI AND ALMONDS

- Prep Time: 15 minutes
- Cook Time: 30 minutes
- Serving Size: 4 servings

INGREDIENTS:

- 1 cup wild rice, washed
- 3 cups vegetable broth
- 1 head broccoli, cut into florets
- 1/4 cup chopped almonds
- Salt and pepper to taste

INSTRUCTIONS:

1. In a large saucepan, bring the vegetable broth to a boil.
2. Add the wild rice and lower heat to low.
3. Simmer for 45 minutes, or until the wild rice is soft.

4. Add the broccoli and simmer for 5 minutes longer, or until tender-crisp.

5. Stir in the almonds and season with salt and pepper to taste.

6. Serve hot.

ROASTED CAULIFLOWER WEDGES

- Prep Time: 15 minutes
- Cook Time: 25 minutes
- Serving Size: 4 servings

INGREDIENTS:

- 1 head cauliflower, cut into wedges
- 2 tablespoons olive oil
- Salt and pepper to taste

INSTRUCTIONS:

1. Preheat oven to 400 degrees F (200 degrees C).

2. Toss the cauliflower wedges with olive oil, salt, and pepper.

3. Spread the cauliflower wedges in a single layer on a baking pan.

4. Roast for 25 minutes, or until the cauliflower is soft and slightly browned.

ROASTED BEETS WITH ORANGE SAUCE AND OLIVES

- Prep Time: 20 minutes
- Cook Time: 45 minutes
- Serving Size: 4 servings

INGREDIENTS:

- 4 medium beets, washed and trimmed
- 2 tablespoons olive oil
- Salt and pepper to taste
- 1/4 cup orange juice
- 2 tablespoons balsamic vinegar
- 1/4 cup chopped Kalamata olives

INSTRUCTIONS:

1. Preheat oven to 400 degrees F (200 degrees C).

2. Wrap the beets in aluminum foil and roast for 45 minutes, or until tender.

3. Unwrap the beets and let them cool somewhat.

4. Cut the beets into wedges and mix them with olive oil, salt, and pepper.

5. In a small bowl, mix together the orange juice and balsamic vinegar.

6. Pour the orange sauce over the beets and top with olives.

7. Serve heated or at room temperature.

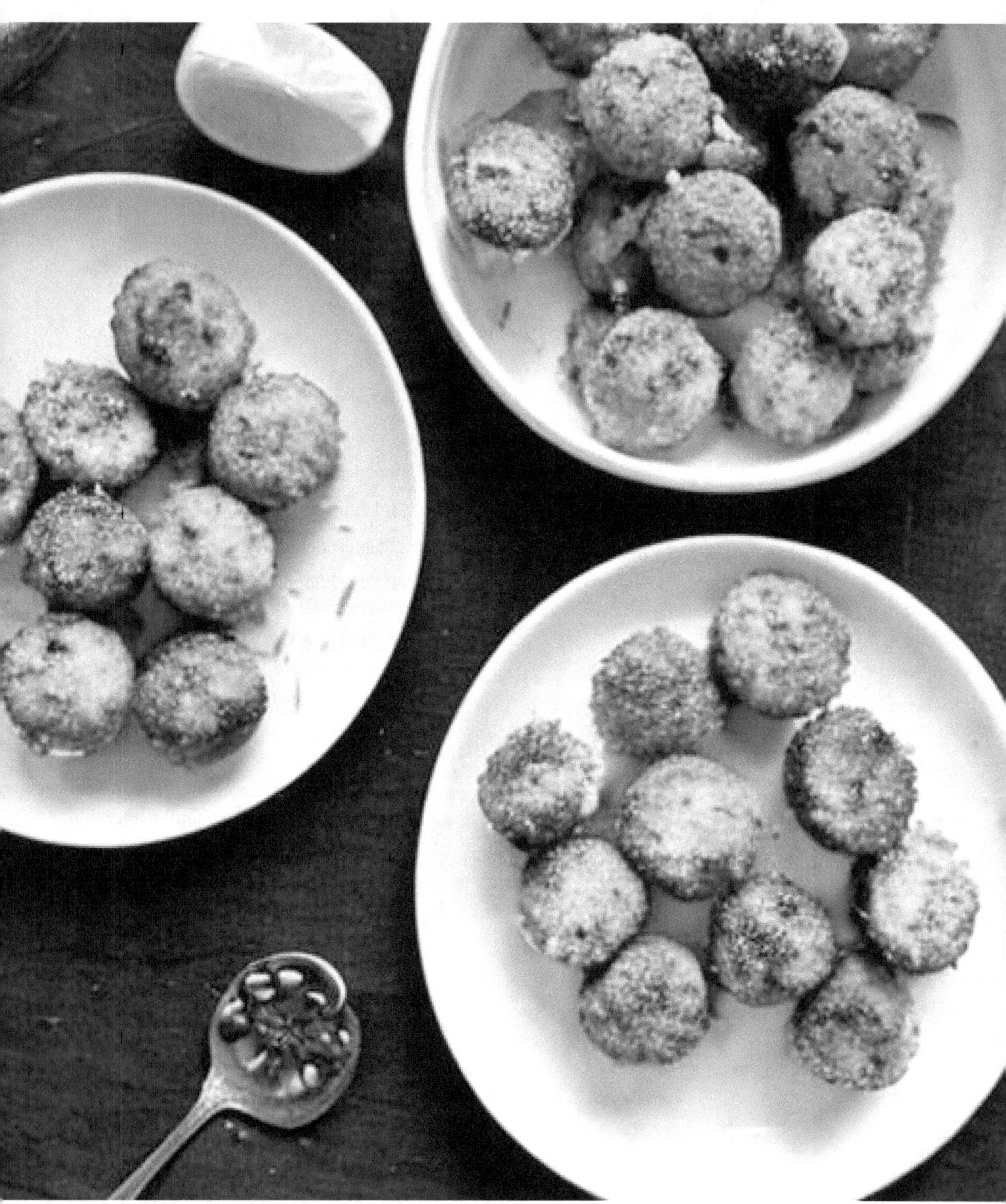

CHEESECAKE DIP

- Prep time: 10 minutes
- Cooking time: None
- Serving size: 4 servings

NUTRITIONAL VALUES:

- Calories: 250
- Fat: 20 grams
- Protein: 5 grams
- Carbohydrates: 20 grams
- Fiber: 1 gram

INGREDIENTS:

- 8 ounces' cream cheese, softened
- 1/4 cup powdered sugar
- 1 teaspoon vanilla extract
- 1/4 cup graham cracker crumbs

INSTRUCTIONS:

1. In a medium bowl, mix together the cream cheese, powdered sugar, and vanilla extract until smooth.
2. Fold in the graham cracker crumbs until completely mixed.
3. Serve with fresh fruit, crackers, or pretzels.

TAHINI AND SEEDS GRANOLA BARS

- Prep time: 15 minutes
- Cooking time: 20 minutes
- Serving size: 12 bars

NUTRITIONAL VALUES:

- Calories: 200
- Fat: 10 grams
- Protein: 5 grams
- Carbohydrates: 30 grams
- Fiber: 5 grams

INGREDIENTS:

- 1 cup rolled oats
- 1/2 cup almond flour
- 1/4 cup tahini
- 1/4 cup maple syrup
- 1/4 cup honey
- 1 teaspoon vanilla extract
- 1/4 cup mixed nuts and seeds (such as almonds, walnuts, sunflower seeds, and pumpkin seeds)

INSTRUCTIONS:

1. Preheat oven to 350 degrees F (175 degrees C). Line a baking sheet with parchment paper.

2. In a large bowl, mix the oats, almond flour, tahini, maple syrup, honey, and vanilla extract.

3. Stir in the mixed nuts and seeds.

4. Spread the mixture evenly on the prepared baking sheet.

5. Bake for 20 minutes, or until golden brown.

6. Let the granola cool fully before cutting into bars.

TOFU NUGGETS

- Prep time: 15 minutes
- Cooking time: 20 minutes
- Serving size: 4 servings

NUTRITIONAL VALUES:

- Calories: 200
- Fat: 10 grams
- Protein: 20 grams
- Carbohydrates: 15 grams
- Fiber: 5 grams

INGREDIENTS:

- 1 block extra-firm tofu, drained and pressed
- 1/2 cup all-purpose flour
- 1 teaspoon baking powder
- 1/2 teaspoon salt
- 1/4 teaspoon black pepper
- 1/4 cup vegan bread crumbs
- 1/4 cup olive oil

INSTRUCTIONS:

1. Crumble the tofu into a medium basin.

2. In a separate basin, mix together the flour, baking powder, salt, and pepper.

3. Add the flour mixture to the tofu and stir until fully blended.

4. Form the tofu mixture into 12 nuggets.

5. Dip the nuggets in the bread crumbs.

6. Heat the olive oil in a large pan over medium heat.

7. Cook the nuggets for 5-7 minutes each side, or until golden brown.

8. Serve with your favorite dipping sauce.

SPICED PECANS

- Prep time: 10 minutes
- Cooking time: 15 minutes
- Serving size: 1 cup

NUTRITIONAL VALUES:

- Calories: 300
- Fat: 25 grams
- Protein: 5 grams
- Carbohydrates: 15 grams
- Fiber: 3 grams

INGREDIENTS:

- 1 cup pecan halves

- 1 tablespoon olive oil
- 1 teaspoon chili powder
- 1/2 teaspoon smoked paprika
- 1/4 teaspoon salt
- 1/4 teaspoon black pepper

INSTRUCTIONS:

1. Preheat oven to 350 degrees F (175 degrees C). Line a baking sheet with parchment paper.
2. Toss the pecans with the olive oil, chile powder, smoked paprika, salt, and pepper.
3. Spread the pecans in a single layer on the prepared baking sheet.
4. Bake for 15 minutes, or until the pecans are aromatic and slightly browned.
5. Let the pecans cool fully before storing in an airtight container.

SMOKY TEMPEH-STUFFED MUSHROOMS

- **Prep time: 20 minutes**
- **Cooking time: 25 minutes**
- **Serving size: 4 servings**

NUTRITIONAL VALUES:

- Calories: 250
- Fat: 15 grams
- Protein: 20 grams
- Carbohydrates: 20 grams
- Fiber: 5 grams

INGREDIENTS:

- 4 huge Portobello mushrooms, brushed clean
- 1 tablespoon olive oil
- 1 onion, chopped
- 2 cloves garlic, minced
- 1/2 cup cooked crumbled tempeh
- 1/4 cup chopped fresh parsley
- 1 tablespoon smoked paprika
- 1/2 teaspoon salt
- 1/4 teaspoon black pepper
- 1/4 cup grated vegan Parmesan cheese

INSTRUCTIONS:

1. Preheat oven to 400 degrees F (200 degrees C).
2. Remove the stems from the Portobello mushrooms and discard.
3. In a large skillet, heat the olive oil over medium heat.
4. Add the onion and simmer until softened, approximately 5 minutes.
5. Add the garlic and simmer for 1 minute longer.
6. Add the cooked tempeh, parsley, smoked paprika, salt, and pepper.
7. Stir well to mix.

8. Spoon the tempeh mixture into the Portobello mushroom caps.

9. Sprinkle with grated vegan Parmesan cheese.

10. Place the filled mushrooms on a baking sheet and bake for 20 minutes, or until the mushrooms are soft and the cheese is melted.

11. Serve hot.

Tips:

1. For an additional Smokey taste, use liquid smoke in lieu of olive oil.

2. If you don't have tempeh, you may use crumbled tofu instead.

3. You may also add additional veggies to the filling, such as diced bell peppers or carrots.

CANDIED COCONUT CASHEWS

- Prep time: 10 minutes
- Cooking time: 20 minutes
- Serving size: 1 cup

NUTRITIONAL VALUES:

- Calories: 300
- Fat: 20 grams
- Protein: 5 grams
- Carbohydrates: 35 grams
- Fiber: 3 grams

INGREDIENTS:

- 1 cup cashews
- 1/4 cup granulated sugar
- 1/4 cup unsweetened shredded coconut
- 1 teaspoon vanilla extract

INSTRUCTIONS:

1. Preheat oven to 350 degrees F (175 degrees C). Line a baking sheet with parchment paper.

2. In a large bowl, mix the cashews, sugar, coconut, and vanilla essence.

3. Toss to coat the cashews evenly.

4. Spread the cashews in a single layer on the prepared baking sheet.

5. Bake for 20 minutes, or until the cashews are golden brown and the coconut is toasted.

6. Let the cashews cool fully before storing in an airtight container.

PANKO JALAPEÑO POPPERS

- Prep time: 15 minutes
- Cooking time: 15 minutes
- Serving size: 12 poppers

NUTRITIONAL VALUES:

- Calories: 200
- Fat: 10 grams
- Protein: 5 grams
- Carbohydrates: 25 grams
- Fiber: 2 grams

INGREDIENTS:

- 12 jalapeño peppers, halves and seeded
- 1/2 cup cream cheese, softened
- 1/4 cup shredded cheddar cheese
- 1/4 cup panko bread crumbs
- 1 teaspoon olive oil

INSTRUCTIONS:

1. Preheat oven to 400 degrees F (200 degrees C). Line a baking sheet with parchment paper.
2. In a medium bowl, mix the cream cheese, cheddar cheese, panko bread crumbs, and olive oil.
3. Stuff the jalapeño pepper halves with the cream cheese mixture.
4. Place the filled peppers on the prepared baking sheet.
5. Bake for 15 minutes, or until the peppers are soft and the cheese has melted.
6. Serve hot.

Tips:

1. For a hotter popper, leave some seeds in the jalapeño peppers.
2. You may also add additional ingredients to the cream cheese mixture, such as chopped bacon or sliced bell peppers.
3. If you desire a crispy exterior, you may fry the jalapeño poppers instead of baking them. Simply heat some oil in a pan over medium heat and cook the poppers for 2-3 minutes each side, or until golden brown.

BAKED BRIE WITH APRICOT-WALNUT JAM

- **Prep time: 15 minutes**
- **Cooking time: 20 minutes**
- **Serving time: 5 minutes**
- **Total time: 40 minutes**

NUTRITIONAL VALUES PER SERVING:

- Calories: 350
- Fat: 25 grams
- Protein: 10 grams
- Carbohydrates: 30 grams
- Fiber: 2 grams

INGREDIENTS:

- 8 ounces Brie cheese, rind removed
- 1/2 cup apricot preserves
- 1/4 cup chopped walnuts
- 1 tablespoon olive oil
- Salt and pepper to taste

INSTRUCTIONS:

1. Preheat oven to 375°F (190°C).
2. In a small dish, mix the apricot preserves and walnuts.
3. Place the Brie cheese on a baking sheet lined with parchment paper.
4. Spread the apricot-walnut mixture evenly over the top of the Brie cheese.
5. Drizzle with olive oil and season with salt and pepper to taste.
6. Bake for 15-20 minutes, or until the Brie cheese is melted and bubbling.
7. Let the Brie cheese sit for 5 minutes before serving.

Tips:

1. For a sweeter taste, add honey or maple syrup instead of apricot preserves.
2. You may also add additional nuts, such as pecans or almonds, to the apricot-walnut combination.
3. Serve the Baked Brie with Apricot-Walnut Jam with crackers, crostini, or sliced fruit.

BRUSCHETTA WITH ROASTED TOMATOES AND BASIL

- Prep time: 15 minutes
- Cooking time: 20 minutes
- Serving time: 5 minutes
- Total time: 40 minutes

NUTRITIONAL VALUES PER SERVING:

- Calories: 150
- Fat: 10 grams
- Protein: 5 grams
- Carbohydrates: 20 grams
- Fiber: 2 grams

INGREDIENTS:

- 1 baguette, sliced
- 2 tablespoons olive oil
- 2 cups cherry tomatoes, halved
- 1/4 cup chopped fresh basil
- 1 clove garlic, minced
- Salt and pepper to taste

INSTRUCTIONS:

1. Preheat oven to 400°F (200°C).
2. Toss the cherry tomatoes with olive oil, garlic, salt, and pepper.

3. Spread the tomatoes on a baking sheet lined with parchment paper.

4. Roast for 20 minutes, or until the tomatoes are soft and slightly caramelized.

5. Top each baguette slice with a tablespoon of roasted tomatoes.

6. Garnish with chopped basil.

7. Serve immediately.

Tips:

1. For a more delicious bruschetta, marinate the tomatoes in the olive oil, garlic, salt, and pepper for 30 minutes before roasting.

2. You may also add additional toppings to the bruschetta, such as sliced mozzarella cheese or anchovies.

3. Serve the Bruschetta with Roasted Tomatoes and Basil as an appetizer or a light snack.

MINI QUICHES WITH SWISS CHEESE AND BACON

- **Prep time: 20 minutes**
- **Cooking time: 30 minutes**
- **Serving time: 10 minutes**
- **Total time: 60 minutes**

NUTRITIONAL VALUES PER SERVING:

- Calories: 250
- Fat: 15 grams
- Protein: 10 grams
- Carbohydrates: 25 grams
- Fiber: 2 grams

INGREDIENTS:

- 12 tiny pie crusts
- 1/4 cup chopped cooked bacon
- 1/2 cup shredded Swiss cheese
- 2 eggs
- 1/2 cup milk
- 1/4 teaspoon salt
- 1/4 teaspoon black pepper

INSTRUCTIONS:

1. Preheat oven to 350°F (175°C).

2. Divide the cooked bacon and grated Swiss cheese equally among the small pie crusts.

3. In a medium bowl, mix together the eggs, milk, salt, and pepper.

4. Pour the egg mixture equally over the bacon and Swiss cheese in the tiny pie crusts.

5. Bake for 20-25 minutes, or until the eggs are set and the crusts are golden brown.

6. Let the quiches cool for 5-10 minutes before serving.

1. For a fuller taste, try a blend of Swiss cheese and cheddar cheese.
2. You may also add additional components to the quiches, such as chopped veggies or cooked sausage.
3. Serve the Mini

SALMON CROSTINI WITH CAPERS AND LEMON

- Prep time: 15 minutes
- Cooking time: 10 minutes
- Serving time: 5 minutes
- Total time: 30 minutes

NUTRITIONAL VALUES PER SERVING:

- Calories: 150
- Fat: 10 grams
- Protein: 15 grams
- Carbohydrates: 10 grams
- Fiber: 1 gram

INGREDIENTS:

- 8 slices baguette, toasted
- 4 ounces smoked salmon, flakes
- 1/4 cup capers, drained
- 2 teaspoons lemon juice
- 1 tablespoon olive oil
- Salt and pepper to taste

INSTRUCTIONS:

1. In a small bowl, mix the smoked salmon, capers, lemon juice, and olive oil.
2. Season with salt and pepper to taste.
3. Spread the salmon mixture equally over the toasted baguette pieces.
4. Serve immediately.

Tips:

1. For a deeper taste, add cream cheese instead of olive oil.
2. You may also add additional toppings to the crostini, such as chopped fresh herbs or a sprinkling of red pepper flakes.

SPRING ROLLS WITH VEGETABLES AND PEANUT SAUCE

- Prep time: 20 minutes
- Cooking time: 10 minutes
- Serving time: 5 minutes
- Total time: 35 minutes

NUTRITIONAL VALUES PER SERVING:

- Calories: 200
- Fat: 15 grams

- Protein: 5 grams
- Carbohydrates: 25 grams
- Fiber: 3 grams

INGREDIENTS:

- 12 rice paper wrappers
- 1 cup shredded carrots
- 1 cup shredded cucumber
- 1/2 cup shredded red bell pepper
- 1/4 cup chopped fresh cilantro
- 1/4 cup peanut sauce

INSTRUCTIONS:

1. Fill a small dish with warm water.
2. Dip one rice paper wrapper in the water until it is soft and flexible.
3. Lay the softened rice paper wrapper on a flat surface.
4. Top the rice paper wrapper with a tiny quantity of shredded carrots, cucumber, red bell pepper, and cilantro.
5. Roll the rice paper wrapper securely from one end to the other.
6. Repeat steps 2-5 with the remaining rice paper wrappers and veggies.
7. To serve, split the spring rolls in half and put them on a dish.
8. Serve with peanut sauce for dipping.

1. For a savory filling, add cooked shrimp or tofu to the veggies.
2. You may also use different kinds of vegetables, such as shredded cabbage or lettuce.
3. If you don't have peanut sauce, you may substitute a store-bought sweet and sour sauce or a soy-based dipping sauce.

ROASTED CHICKPEAS

- **Prep time: 10 minutes**
- **Cooking time: 30 minutes**
- **Serving time: 5 minutes**
- **Total time: 45 minutes**

NUTRITIONAL VALUES PER SERVING:

- Calories: 200
- Fat: 12 grams
- Protein: 10 grams
- Carbohydrates: 25 grams
- Fiber: 5 grams

INGREDIENTS:

- 1 can (15 ounces) chickpeas, drained and rinsed
- 1 tablespoon olive oil
- 1 teaspoon smoked paprika
- 1/2 teaspoon salt
- 1/4 teaspoon black pepper

INSTRUCTIONS:

1. Preheat oven to 400 degrees F (200 degrees C).
2. Toss the chickpeas with olive oil, smoked paprika, salt, and pepper.
3. Spread the chickpeas in a single layer on a baking sheet.
4. Roast for 30 minutes, or until the chickpeas are crispy and golden brown.
5. Serve immediately.

Tips:

1. For a hotter snack, add a sprinkle of cayenne pepper to the chickpeas before roasting.
2. You may also add additional ingredients to the chickpeas, such as cumin or garlic powder.

APPLE SLICES WITH PEANUT BUTTER AND HONEY

- Prep time: 5 minutes
- Cooking time: None
- Serving time: 5 minutes
- Total time: 10 minutes

NUTRITIONAL VALUES PER SERVING:

- Calories: 200
- Fat: 10 grams
- Protein: 5 grams
- Carbohydrates: 30 grams
- Fiber: 3 grams

INGREDIENTS:

- 1 apple, sliced
- 2 tbsp peanut butter
- 1 tablespoon honey

INSTRUCTIONS:

1. Spread peanut butter on each apple slice.
2. Drizzle with honey.
3. Serve immediately.

Tips:

1. For a crunchier snack, try celery sticks or carrot sticks instead of apple slices.
2. You may also use almond butter or cashew butter instead of peanut butter.

TRAIL MIX WITH NUTS, SEEDS, AND DRIED FRUIT

- Prep time: 10 minutes
- Cooking time: None
- Serving time: 5 minutes
- Total time: 15 minutes

NUTRITIONAL VALUES PER SERVING:

- Calories: 200
- Fat: 15 grams
- Protein: 5 grams
- Carbohydrates: 25 grams
- Fiber: 3 grams

INGREDIENTS:

- 1/2 cup mixed nuts (such as almonds, walnuts, and pecans)
- 1/4 cup mixed seeds (such as sunflower seeds, pumpkin seeds, and chia seeds)
- 1/4 cup dried fruit (such as raisins, cranberries, and apricots)

INSTRUCTIONS:

1. Combine the nuts, seeds, and dried fruit in a basin.
2. Toss to coat.
3. Store in an airtight jar at room temperature for up to 2 weeks.

Tips:

1. For a savory trail mix, add a sprinkle of cinnamon or nutmeg.
2. You may also add additional components to the trail mix, such as dark chocolate chips or coconut flakes.

ENERGY BITES

- Prep time: 15 minutes
- Cooking time: None
- Serving time: 5 minutes
- Total time: 20 minutes

NUTRITIONAL VALUES PER SERVING:

- Calories: 200
- Fat: 10 grams
- Protein: 5 grams
- Carbohydrates: 30 grams
- Fiber: 3 grams

INGREDIENTS:

- 1 cup rolled oats

- 1/2 cup almond butter
- 1/4 cup honey
- 1/4 cup tiny chocolate chips
- 1/4 cup chopped dried fruit (such as raisins, cranberries, or apricots)

INSTRUCTIONS:

1. In a large bowl, mix the rolled oats, almond butter, honey, chocolate chips, and dried fruit.
2. Mix vigorously until the ingredients are uniformly distributed.
3. Roll the mixture into balls.
4. Store in an airtight jar in the refrigerator for up to 2 weeks.

Tips:

1. For a savory energy bite, add a sprinkle of cinnamon or nutmeg.
2. You may also add additional components to the energy bites, such as almonds, seeds, or coconut flakes.

GOBI MANCHURIAN

- Prep time: 20 minutes
- Cooking time: 30 minutes
- Serving time: 10 minutes
- Total time: 60 minutes

NUTRITIONAL VALUES PER SERVING:

- Calories: 300
- Fat: 10 grams
- Protein: 15 grams
- Carbohydrates: 40 grams
- Fiber: 5 grams

INGREDIENTS:

- 1 head cauliflower, cut into florets
- 1/2 cup cornstarch
- 1 tablespoon soy sauce
- 1 tablespoon rice vinegar
- 1 tablespoon vegetable oil
- 1 tablespoon ginger, grated
- 2 cloves garlic, minced
- 1 onion, chopped
- 1 red bell pepper, chopped 1 green bell pepper, chopped 1/2 cup Manchurian sauce

INSTRUCTIONS:

1. In a large dish, mix the cauliflower florets with the cornstarch until equally coated.
2. Heat the vegetable oil in a large wok or pan over medium-high heat.
3. Add the cauliflower florets and heat until golden brown and crispy, approximately 5 minutes.
4. Remove the cauliflower from the pan and put aside.
5. In the same wok, add the ginger, garlic, onion, red bell pepper, and green bell pepper.
6. Cook until the veggies are tender-crisp, approximately 5 minutes.
7. Stir in the Manchurian sauce and bring to a boil.
8. Return the cooked cauliflower florets to the skillet and toss to cover with the sauce.
9. Serve immediately over rice or noodles.

Tips:

1. For a hotter meal, add a sprinkle of cayenne pepper to the Manchurian sauce.
2. You may also add additional veggies to the meal, such as carrots or broccoli.

3. Store the Gobi Manchurian in an airtight container in the refrigerator for up to 2 days.

CAULIFLOWER AND SWEET POTATO CRUST PIZZAS

- Prep time: 30 minutes
- Cooking time: 20 minutes
- Serving time: 10 minutes
- Total time: 60 minutes

NUTRITIONAL VALUES PER SERVING:

- Calories: 400
- Fat: 15 grams
- Protein: 15 grams
- Carbohydrates: 50 grams
- Fiber: 5 grams

INGREDIENTS:

For the crust:

- 1 head cauliflower, grated
- 1 sweet potato, grated
- 1/2 cup almond flour
- 1/4 cup nutritional yeast
- 1 teaspoon dried oregano
- 1/2 teaspoon salt
- 1/4 teaspoon black pepper

For the toppings:

- 1/2 cup vegan pizza sauce
- 1 cup shredded vegan cheese
- 1/2 cup chopped veggies (optional)

INSTRUCTIONS:

1. Preheat oven to 400 degrees F (200 degrees C).
2. In a large bowl, mix the grated cauliflower, grated sweet potato, almond flour, nutritional yeast, dried oregano, salt, and pepper.
3. Mix vigorously until the ingredients are uniformly distributed.
4. Press the mixture into two 12-inch pizza crusts on baking pans.
5. Spread the pizza sauce over each pizza dough.
6. Top with the shredded vegan cheese and chopped veggies (if using).
7. Bake for 20 minutes, or until the crust is golden brown and the cheese has melted.
8. Serve immediately.

Tips:

1. For a deeper taste, use full-fat coconut milk instead of almond milk in the pizza sauce.
2. You may also add additional veggies to the pizzas, such as bell peppers, mushrooms, or olives.

3. Store the Cauliflower and Sweet Potato Crust Pizzas in an airtight container in the refrigerator for up to 3 days.

SWEET POTATO AND BLACK BEAN EMPANADAS

- Prep time: 20 minutes
- Cooking time: 30 minutes
- Serving time: 10 minutes
- Total time: 60 minutes

NUTRITIONAL VALUES PER SERVING:

- Calories: 300
- Fat: 10 grams
- Protein: 15 grams
- Carbohydrates: 40 grams
- Fiber: 5 grams

INGREDIENTS:

For the filling:

- 1 tablespoon olive oil
- 1 onion, chopped
- 1 clove garlic, minced
- 1 cup cooked mashed sweet potato
- 1 cup cooked black beans, rinsed and drained
- 1/2 cup sliced bell peppers
- 1/4 cup chopped cilantro
- 1 teaspoon cumin
- 1/2 teaspoon chili powder
- 1/4 teaspoon salt
- 1/4 teaspoon black pepper

For the dough:

- 1 1/2 cups all-purpose flour
- 1 teaspoon baking powder
- 1/2 teaspoon salt
- 1/2 cup chilled vegan butter, cut into cubes
- 1/4 cup cold water
- 1 tablespoon cider vinegar

INSTRUCTIONS:

Make the filling: In a large bowl, mix the olive oil, onion, and garlic. Cook over medium heat until softened, approximately 5 minutes. Stir in the mashed sweet potato, black beans, bell peppers, cilantro, cumin, chili powder, salt, and pepper. Mix vigorously until the ingredients are uniformly distributed. Set aside to cool.

Make the dough: In a large bowl, mix together the flour and baking powder. Cut in the vegan butter with a pastry cutter or two knives until the mixture resembles coarse crumbs. Stir in the cold water and vinegar until the dough almost comes together. Form the dough into a disk, cover in plastic wrap, and chill for at least 30 minutes.

1. Preheat oven to 375 degrees F (190 degrees C).

2. Roll out the dough on a lightly floured surface to approximately 1/8-inch thickness. Cut out 3-inch circles using a cookie cutter or the rim of a glass.

3. Place a dollop of the filling in the middle of each dough round. Fold the dough over in half and crimp the edges with a fork to seal.

4. Place the empanadas on a baking sheet lined with parchment paper.

5. Bake for 20-25 minutes, or until the empanadas are golden brown.

6. Serve immediately with your favorite dipping sauce.

Tips:

1. For a hotter empanada, add a sprinkle of cayenne pepper to the filling.

2. You may also add additional veggies to the mixture, such as corn or zucchini.

3. Store the Sweet Potato and Black Bean Empanadas in an airtight container in the refrigerator for up to 3 days.

DECONSTRUCTED SUSHI BOWLS

NUTRITIONAL VALUES PER SERVING:

- Calories: 400
- Fat: 15 grams
- Protein: 20 grams
- Carbohydrates: 55 grams
- Fiber: 5 grams

INGREDIENTS:

- 1 cup cooked brown rice
- 1 cup cooked edamame
- 1/2 cup sliced carrots
- 1/2 cup chopped cucumbers
- 1/4 cup chopped avocado
- 1/4 cup chopped mango
- 2 teaspoons soy sauce
- 1 tablespoon rice vinegar
- 1 tablespoon sesame oil
- 1 teaspoon wasabi (optional)
- 1 tablespoon shredded nori (optional)

INSTRUCTIONS:

1. In a large bowl, add the cooked brown rice, cooked edamame, chopped carrots, diced cucumbers, chopped avocado, and chopped mango.

2. In a small bowl, mix together the soy sauce, rice vinegar, and sesame oil.

3. Pour the sauce over the rice and veggie mixture and toss to coat.

4. If using wasabi, add a little amount to each bowl and swirl to distribute equally.

5. Top with shredded nori, if desired.

6. Serve immediately.

1. For a hotter dish, add a sprinkle of cayenne pepper to the sauce.

2. You may also add additional veggies to the dish, such as bell peppers, zucchini, or mushrooms.

3. Store the Deconstructed Sushi Bowls in an airtight container in the refrigerator for up to 2 days.

ZUCCHINI LASAGNA POCKETS

NUTRITIONAL VALUES PER SERVING:

- Calories: 350
- Fat: 15 grams
- Protein: 15 grams
- Carbohydrates: 40 grams
- Fiber: 5 grams

INGREDIENTS:

For the filling:

- 1 tablespoon olive oil
- 1 onion, chopped
- 2 cloves garlic, minced
- 1 zucchini, grated
- 1 red bell pepper, chopped
- 1/2 cup chopped mushrooms
- 1 cup spinach, chopped
- 1 (14.5-ounce) can chopped tomatoes, undrained
- 1 tablespoon dried oregano
- 1/2 teaspoon salt
- 1/4 teaspoon black pepper

For the zucchini pockets:

- 2 medium zucchini, halved lengthwise
- 1/2 cup vegan ricotta cheese
- 1/4 cup nutritional yeast
- 1/4 cup chopped fresh parsley

INSTRUCTIONS:

1. Preheat oven to 375 degrees F (190 degrees C).

2. Make the filling: In a large saucepan, heat the olive oil over medium heat.

3. Add the onion and garlic and simmer until softened, approximately 5 minutes.

4. Add the zucchini, red bell pepper, mushrooms, spinach, chopped tomatoes, oregano, salt, and pepper.

5. Bring to a boil and simmer for 15 minutes, or until the veggies are cooked.

6. Remove from heat and put aside to cool.

7. Make the zucchini pockets: In a small bowl, mix the vegan ricotta cheese, nutritional yeast, and parsley.

8. Scoop the ricotta mixture into the middle of each zucchini half.

9. Fill the zucchini halves with the chilled veggie filling.

10. Bake for 20 minutes, or until the zucchini is soft and the mixture is cooked through.

11. Serve immediately.

Tips:

1. For a fuller taste, use full-fat coconut milk instead of almond milk in the filling.

2. You may also add additional veggies to the mixture, such as maize or carrots.

3. Store the Zucchini Lasagna Pockets in an airtight container in the refrigerator for up to 2 days.

SWEET POTATO AND CORN FALAFEL

- **Prep time: 20 minutes**
- **Cook time: 15 minutes**
- **Serving time: 10 minutes**
- **Total time: 45 minutes**

NUTRITIONAL VALUES PER SERVING:

- Calories: 250
- Fat: 10 grams
- Protein: 10 grams
- Carbohydrates: 30 grams
- Fiber: 5 grams

INGREDIENTS:

- 1 medium sweet potato, boiled and mashed
- 1/2 cup cooked corn kernels
- 1/4 cup chopped onion
- 1/4 cup chopped cilantro
- 1 tablespoon olive oil
- 2 cloves garlic, minced
- 1 teaspoon cumin
- 1/2 teaspoon smoked paprika
- 1/4 teaspoon salt
- 1/4 teaspoon black pepper

INSTRUCTIONS:

1. In a large bowl, mix the mashed sweet potato, cooked corn kernels, chopped onion, chopped cilantro, olive oil, garlic, cumin, smoked paprika, salt, and pepper.

2. Mix vigorously until the ingredients are uniformly distributed.

3. Form the mixture into 4-6 patties.

4. Heat a large skillet over medium heat.

5. Cook the patties for 5-7 minutes each side, or until they are golden brown and cooked through.

6. Serve on buns with your preferred toppings.

Tips:

1. For a heartier burger, add 1/4 cup of rolled oats to the mixture.

2. You may also add additional veggies to the patties, such as bell peppers or zucchini.

3. Store the Sweet Potato and Corn Falafel in an airtight container in the refrigerator for up to 3 days.

PIZZA BOATS WITH EGGPLANT AND CHICKPEAS

- Prep time: 20 minutes
- Cooking time: 25 minutes
- Serving time: 10 minutes
- Total time: 55 minutes

NUTRITIONAL VALUES PER SERVING:

- Calories: 350
- Fat: 15 grams
- Protein: 15 grams
- Carbohydrates: 40 grams
- Fiber: 5 grams

INGREDIENTS:

- 2 medium eggplant, halved lengthwise
- 1 tablespoon olive oil
- 1 onion, chopped
- 2 cloves garlic, minced
- 1 (14.5-ounce) can chopped tomatoes, undrained
- 1/2 cup cooked chickpeas, rinsed and drained
- 1/4 cup chopped basil
- 1 tablespoon dried oregano
- 1/2 teaspoon salt
- 1/4 teaspoon black pepper

INSTRUCTIONS:

1. Preheat oven to 375 degrees F (190 degrees C).

2. Score the flesh of each eggplant half in a crosshatch pattern.

3. Drizzle the eggplant halves with olive oil and sprinkle with salt and pepper.

4. Place the eggplant halves on a baking pan and bake for 15 minutes, or until soft.

5. While the eggplant is roasting, heat the olive oil in a large pan over medium heat.

6. Add the onion and garlic and simmer until softened, approximately 5 minutes.

7. Stir in the diced tomatoes, chickpeas, chopped basil, dry oregano, salt, and pepper.

8. Bring to a boil and simmer for 10 minutes, or until the sauce has thickened.

9. Remove the eggplant halves from the oven and ladle the sauce into each half.

10. Bake for a further 10 minutes, or until the eggplant is cooked through.

11. Serve immediately.

Tips:

1. For a hotter pizza boat, add a sprinkle of cayenne pepper to the sauce.

2. You may also add additional veggies to the sauce, such as zucchini or bell peppers.

3. Store the Pizza Boats with Eggplant and Chickpeas in an airtight container in the refrigerator for up to 2 days.

BANG BANG "SHRIMP"

- Prep time: 20 minutes
- Cooking time: 15 minutes
- Serving time: 10 minutes
- Total time: 45 minutes

NUTRITIONAL VALUES PER SERVING:

- Calories: 300
- Fat: 10 grams
- Protein: 15 grams
- Carbohydrates: 40 grams
- Fiber: 5 grams

INGREDIENTS:

- 1 package cauliflower florets, sliced into bite-sized portions
- 1/4 cup cornstarch
- 1/2 teaspoon salt
- 1/4 teaspoon black pepper
- 1 tablespoon vegetable oil

For the sauce:

- 1/4 cup vegan mayonnaise
- 1 tablespoon Sriracha sauce
- 1 tablespoon sweet chili sauce
- 1 tablespoon rice vinegar
- 1 teaspoon sesame oil
- 1 clove garlic, minced

INSTRUCTIONS:

1. In a large basin, mix the cauliflower florets with the cornstarch, salt, and pepper until equally covered.

2. Heat the vegetable oil in a large pan or wok over medium-high heat.

3. Add the cauliflower florets and heat until golden brown and crispy, approximately 5 minutes.

4. In a small bowl, mix together the vegan mayonnaise, Sriracha sauce, sweet chili sauce, rice vinegar, sesame oil, and garlic until smooth.

5. Pour the sauce over the cooked cauliflower florets and toss to coat.

6. Serve immediately over rice or noodles.

Tips:

1. For a hotter meal, add extra Sriracha sauce to the taste.

2. You may also add additional veggies to the recipe, such as broccoli or bell peppers.

3. Store the Bang Bang "Shrimp" in an airtight container in the refrigerator for up to 3 days.

ZUCCHINI LASAGNA POCKETS

- **Prep time: 20 minutes**
- **Cooking time: 20 minutes**
- **Serving time: 10 minutes**
- **Total time: 50 minutes**

NUTRITIONAL VALUES PER SERVING:

- Calories: 350
- Fat: 15 grams
- Protein: 15 grams
- Carbohydrates: 40 grams
- Fiber: 5 grams

INGREDIENTS:

For the filling:

- 1 tablespoon olive oil
- 1 onion, chopped
- 2 cloves garlic, minced
- 1 zucchini, grated
- 1 red bell pepper, chopped
- 1/2 cup chopped mushrooms
- 1 cup spinach, chopped
- 1 (14.5-ounce) can chopped tomatoes, undrained
- 1 tablespoon dried oregano
- 1/2 teaspoon salt
- 1/4 teaspoon black pepper

For the zucchini pockets:

- 2 medium zucchini, halved lengthwise
- 1/2 cup vegan ricotta cheese
- 1/4 cup nutritional yeast
- 1/4 cup chopped fresh parsley

INSTRUCTIONS:

1. Preheat oven to 375 degrees F (190 degrees C).

2. Make the filling: In a large saucepan, heat the olive oil over medium heat.

3. Add the onion and garlic and simmer until softened, approximately 5 minutes.

4. Add the zucchini, red bell pepper, mushrooms, spinach, chopped tomatoes, oregano, salt, and pepper.

5. Bring to a boil and simmer for 15 minutes, or until the veggies are cooked.

6. Remove from heat and put aside to cool.

7. Make the zucchini pockets: In a small bowl, mix the vegan ricotta cheese, nutritional yeast, and parsley.

8. Scoop the ricotta mixture into the middle of each zucchini half.

9. Fill the zucchini halves with the chilled veggie filling.

10. Bake for 20 minutes, or until the zucchini is soft and the mixture is cooked through.

11. Serve immediately.

Tips:

1. For a fuller taste, use full-fat coconut milk instead of almond milk in the filling.

2. You may also add additional veggies to the mixture, such as maize or carrots.

3. Store the Zucchini Lasagna Pockets in an airtight container in the refrigerator for up to 2 days.

TOFU TIKKA MASALA

- Prep time: 20 minutes
- Cooking time: 25 minutes
- Serving time: 10 minutes
- Total time: 55 minutes

NUTRITIONAL VALUES PER SERVING:

- Calories: 400
- Fat: 15 grams
- Protein: 20 grams
- Carbohydrates: 45 grams
- Fiber: 5 grams

INGREDIENTS:

For the marinade:

- 1/2 cup soy sauce
- 1 tablespoon lemon juice
- 1 tablespoon grated ginger
- 1 tablespoon garlic powder
- 1 teaspoon garam masala
- 1/2 teaspoon turmeric powder
- 1/4 teaspoon chili powder
- 1/4 teaspoon salt

For the tofu:

- 1 block (14 ounces) extra-firm tofu, pressed and drained
- 1 tablespoon olive oil

For the sauce:

- 1 tablespoon olive oil
- 1 onion, chopped
- 2 cloves garlic, minced
- 1 tablespoon grated ginger
- 1 tablespoon garam masala
- 1/2 teaspoon turmeric powder
- 1/4 teaspoon chili powder
- 1 (14.5-ounce) can chopped tomatoes, undrained
- 1 (13.5-ounce) can coconut milk
- 1/4 cup chopped cilantro

INSTRUCTIONS:

Make the marinade:

1. In a large bowl, mix together the soy sauce, lemon juice, grated ginger, garlic powder, garam masala, turmeric powder, chili powder, and salt.
2. Add the tofu to the marinade and toss to coat.
3. Marinate the tofu for at least 15 minutes, or up to 2 hours.
4. Preheat oven to 400 degrees F (200 degrees C).
5. Heat the olive oil in a large pan over medium heat.
6. Add the tofu and heat until golden brown and crispy on both sides, approximately 5 minutes each side.
7. Transfer the tofu to a baking sheet and bake for 10 minutes, or until cooked through.
8. While the tofu is baking, create the sauce: In the same pan used to cook the tofu, heat the olive oil over medium heat.
9. Add the onion and simmer until softened, approximately 5 minutes.
10. Add the garlic, ginger, garam masala, turmeric powder, and chili powder.
11. Cook for 1 minute, or until aromatic.
12. Stir in the chopped tomatoes and coconut milk.
13. Bring to a boil, then decrease heat and simmer for 10 minutes, or until the sauce has thickened.
14. Stir in the chopped cilantro.
15. Add the baked tofu to the sauce and toss to coat.
16. Serve over rice or naan bread.

Tips:

1. For a hotter meal, add additional chili powder to the marinade or sauce.
2. You may also add additional veggies to the sauce, such as bell peppers or carrots.

3. Store the Tofu Tikka Masala in an airtight jar in the refrigerator for up to 3 days.

BAKED POPCORN CAULIFLOWER

- Prep time: 10 minutes
- Cooking time: 30 minutes
- Serving time: 10 minutes
- Total time: 50 minutes

NUTRITIONAL VALUES PER SERVING:

- Calories: 200
- Fat: 10 grams
- Protein: 10 grams
- Carbohydrates: 20 grams
- Fiber: 5 grams

INGREDIENTS:

- 1 head cauliflower, cut into florets
- 1 tablespoon olive oil
- 1 teaspoon nutritional yeast
- 1/2 teaspoon dried oregano
- 1/4 teaspoon salt
- 1/4 teaspoon black pepper

INSTRUCTIONS:

1. Preheat oven to 400 degrees F (200 degrees C).

2. In a large dish, mix the cauliflower florets with the olive oil, nutritional yeast, dried oregano, salt, and pepper until equally coated.

3. Spread the cauliflower florets in a single layer on a baking sheet.

4. Bake for 20-30 minutes, or until the cauliflower is golden brown and crispy.

5. Serve immediately.

Tips:

1. For a hotter meal, add a sprinkle of cayenne pepper to the spice mix.

2. You may also add additional spices to the seasoning mix, such as cumin or paprika.

3. Store the Baked Popcorn Cauliflower in an airtight jar in the refrigerator for up to 3 days.

SOY CURL–STUFFED SQUASH

- Prep time: 20 minutes
- Cooking time: 30 minutes
- Serving time: 10 minutes
- Total time: 60 minutes

NUTRITIONAL VALUES PER SERVING:

- Calories: 350
- Fat: 15 grams
- Protein: 15 grams
- Carbohydrates: 40 grams
- Fiber: 5 grams

INGREDIENTS:

- 1 acorn squash, halved and seeded
- 1 tablespoon olive oil
- 1 onion, chopped
- 2 cloves garlic, minced
- 1 package soy curls, crushed
- 1 teaspoon cumin
- 1/2 teaspoon chili powder
- 1/4 teaspoon salt
- 1/4 teaspoon black pepper
- 1/2 cup chopped cilantro
- 1/4 cup chopped tomatoes

INSTRUCTIONS:

1. Preheat oven to 375 degrees F (190 degrees C).
2. Drizzle the acorn squash halves with olive oil and sprinkle with salt and pepper.
3. Place the squash halves on a baking pan and bake for 15 minutes, or until soft.
4. While the squash is roasting, heat the olive oil in a large pan over medium heat.
5. Add the onion and simmer until softened, approximately 5 minutes.
6. Add the garlic and simmer for 1 minute longer, or until fragrant.
7. Add the crushed soy curls, cumin, chili powder, salt, and pepper.
8. Cook for 5 minutes, or until the soy curls are cooked through.
9. Stir in the chopped cilantro and diced tomatoes.
10. Spoon the soy curl mixture into the cooked acorn squash halves.
11. Bake for a further 10 minutes, or until the filling is cooked through.
12. Serve immediately.

Tips:

1. For a hotter meal, add a sprinkle of cayenne pepper to the soy curl mixture.
2. You may also add additional veggies to the soy curl combination, such as bell peppers or zucchini.
3. Store the Soy Curl–Stuffed Squash in an airtight container in the refrigerator for up to 3 days.

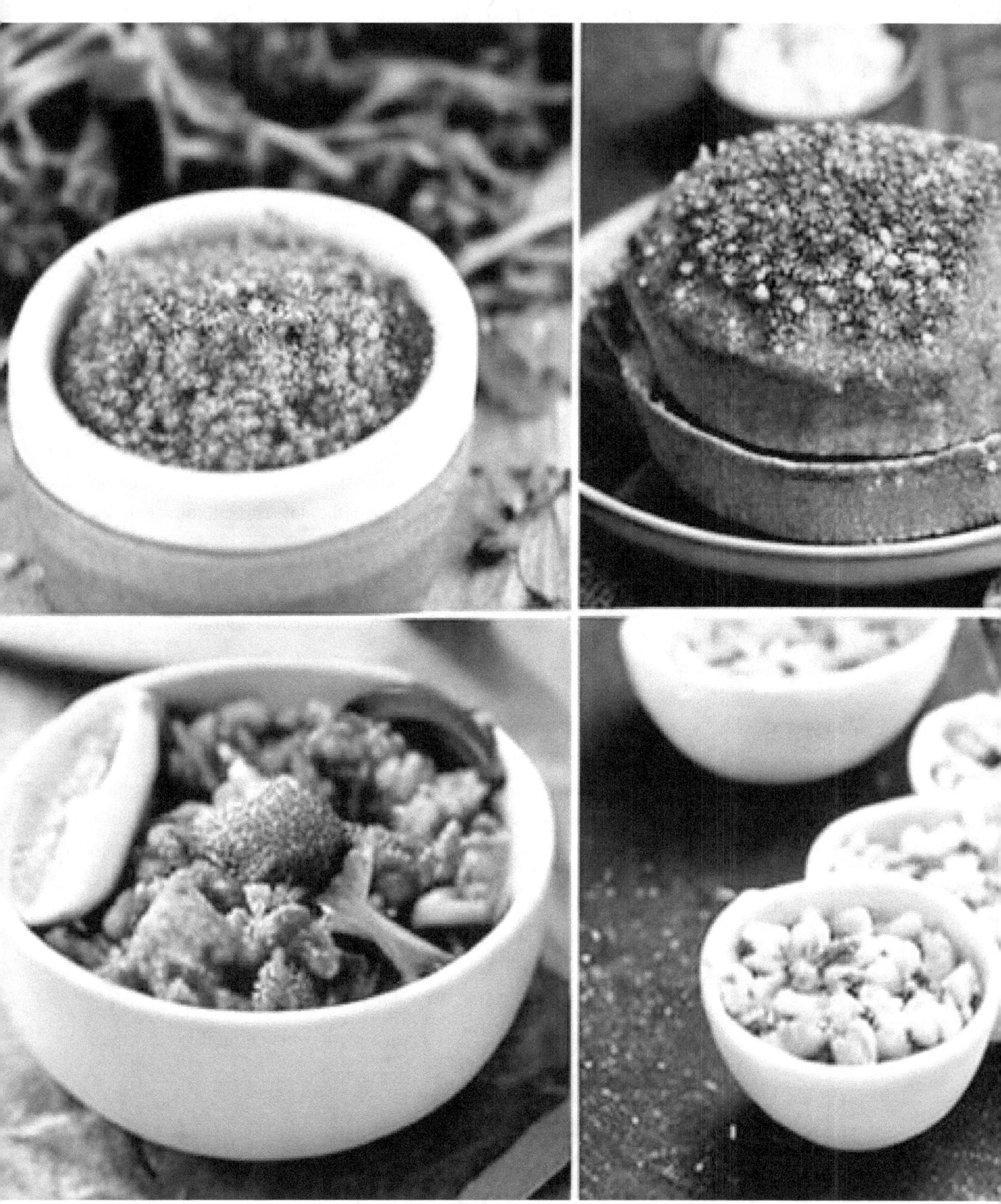

GLUTEN-FREE VEGAN HOMEMADE FLOUR BLEND

- Prep time: 5 minutes
- Cook time: 0 minutes
- Total time: 5 minutes

NUTRITIONAL DATA PER 1/4 CUP (30 GRAMS):

- Calories: 100
- Fat: 3 grams
- Protein: 5 grams
- Carbohydrates: 15 grams
- Fiber: 2 grams

INGREDIENTS:

- 1 cup (120 grams) brown rice flour
- 1/2 cup (60 grams) sorghum flour
- 1/4 cup (50 grams) potato starch
- 1/4 cup (40 grams) tapioca starch
- 1 tablespoon (5 grams) xanthan gum

INSTRUCTIONS:

1. In a large bowl, mix together the brown rice flour, sorghum flour, potato starch, tapioca starch, and xanthan gum until uniformly distributed.
2. Store the flour mix in an airtight container in a cold, dry location.
3. Use the flour mix to prepare your favorite gluten-free vegan dishes.

Tips:

1. For a finer texture, sift the flour mix before using.
2. You may also add additional gluten-free flours to the mix, such as oat flour or millet flour.
3. The gluten-free vegan homemade flour mix may be kept for up to 3 months.

BBQ SAUCE

- Prep time: 10 minutes
- Cook time: 20 minutes
- Total time: 30 minutes

NUTRITIONAL DATA PER 1/4 CUP (60 GRAMS):

- Calories: 100
- Fat: 5 grams
- Protein: 2 grams
- Carbohydrates: 15 grams
- Fiber: 1 gram

INGREDIENTS:

- 1 tablespoon olive oil
- 1 onion, chopped

- 2 cloves garlic, minced
- 1 (14.5-ounce) can chopped tomatoes, undrained
- 1/2 cup unsweetened tomato paste
- 1/4 cup apple cider vinegar
- 1 tablespoon soy sauce
- 1 tablespoon Worcestershire sauce
- 1 tablespoon smoked paprika
- 1 teaspoon chili powder
- 1/2 teaspoon salt
- 1/4 teaspoon black pepper

INSTRUCTIONS:

1. In a large saucepan, heat the olive oil over medium heat.
2. Add the onion and simmer until softened, approximately 5 minutes.
3. Add the garlic and simmer for 1 minute longer, or until fragrant.
4. Add the chopped tomatoes, tomato paste, apple cider vinegar, soy sauce, Worcestershire sauce, smoked paprika, chili powder, salt, and pepper.
5. Bring to a boil, then decrease heat and simmer for 20 minutes, or until the sauce has thickened.
6. Taste and adjust spices as desired.
7. Serve the BBQ sauce over grilled chicken, ribs, or veggies.

Tips:

1. For a hotter BBQ sauce, add a pinch of cayenne pepper.
2. You may also add additional spices to the BBQ sauce, such as cumin or coriander.
3. Store the BBQ sauce in an airtight jar in the refrigerator for up to 2 weeks.

HUMMUS

- Prep time: 15 minutes
- Cook time: 0 minutes
- Total time: 15 minutes

NUTRITIONAL DATA PER 1/4 CUP (60 GRAMS):

- Calories: 200
- Fat: 10 grams
- Protein: 8 grams
- Carbohydrates: 20 grams
- Fiber: 5 grams

INGREDIENTS:

- 1 (15-ounce) can chickpeas, drained and rinsed
- 1/4 cup tahini
- 1/4 cup lemon juice
- 1 clove garlic, minced
- 1 tablespoon olive oil
- 1/4 teaspoon salt
- 1/4 teaspoon cumin powder
- 1/4 teaspoon paprika

🔩 1/4 cup chopped fresh parsley

INSTRUCTIONS:

1. In a food processor, blend the chickpeas, tahini, lemon juice, garlic, olive oil, salt, cumin powder, and paprika.
2. Process until smooth and creamy.
3. Taste and adjust spices as desired.
4. Serve the hummus with pita bread, veggies, or crackers.

Tips:

1. For a smoother hummus, remove the skins from the chickpeas before processing.
2. You may also add additional spices to the hummus, such as coriander or cardamom.
3. Store the hummus in an airtight jar in the refrigerator for up to 5 days.

SUNFLOWER SEED CHEESE SAUCE

🔩 **Prep time: 20 minutes**

🔩 **Cook time: 0 minutes**

🔩 **Total time: 20 minutes**

NUTRITIONAL DATA PER 1/4 CUP (60 GRAMS):

🔩 Calories: 200

🔩 Fat: 15 grams

🔩 Protein: 5 grams

🔩 Carbohydrates: 20 grams

🔩 Fiber: 5 grams

INGREDIENTS:

🔩 1 cup (100 grams) sunflower seeds

🔩 1/2 cup (60 grams) nutritious yeast

🔩 1/4 cup (60 ml) water

🔩 2 teaspoons lemon juice

🔩 1 tablespoon olive oil

🔩 1 clove garlic, minced

🔩 1/2 teaspoon salt

🔩 1/4 teaspoon black pepper

INSTRUCTIONS:

1. In a food processor, blend the sunflower seeds, nutritional yeast, water, lemon juice, olive oil, garlic, salt, and pepper.
2. Process until smooth and creamy.
3. Taste and adjust spices as desired.
4. Serve the sunflower seed cheese sauce over pasta, veggies, or potatoes.

Tips:

1. For a thicker sauce, use full-fat coconut milk instead of water.
2. You may also add additional spices to the sauce, such as nutmeg or paprika.

3. Store the sunflower seed cheese sauce in an airtight jar in the refrigerator for up to 5 days.

CASHEW RANCH DRESSING

- Prep time: 15 minutes
- Cook time: 0 minutes
- Total time: 15 minutes

NUTRITIONAL DATA PER 1/4 CUP (60 GRAMS):

- Calories: 200
- Fat: 10 grams
- Protein: 5 grams
- Carbohydrates: 20 grams
- Fiber: 5 grams

INGREDIENTS:

- 1 cup (120 grams) cashews, soaked for at least 1 hour
- 1/2 cup (120 ml) unsweetened almond milk
- 1/4 cup (60 ml) lemon juice
- 1 tablespoon Dijon mustard
- 1 clove garlic, minced
- 1/2 teaspoon dried dill
- 1/4 teaspoon onion powder
- 1/4 teaspoon salt
- 1/4 teaspoon black pepper

INSTRUCTIONS:

1. In a food processor, blend the soaked cashews, almond milk, lemon juice, Dijon mustard, garlic, dried dill, onion powder, salt, and pepper.
2. Process until smooth and creamy.
3. Taste and adjust spices as desired.
4. Serve the cashew ranch dressing with salads, veggies, or chips.

Tips:

1. For a tangier dressing, add additional lemon juice.
2. You may also add additional herbs and spices to the dressing, such as chives or parsley.
3. Store the cashew ranch dressing in an airtight jar in the refrigerator for up to 5 days.

TEMPEH "BACON"

- Prep time: 10 minutes
- Cook time: 15 minutes
- Total time: 25 minutes

NUTRITIONAL DATA PER 1/4 CUP (30 GRAMS):

- Calories: 100
- Fat: 7 grams
- Protein: 10 grams
- Carbohydrates: 5 grams
- Fiber: 2 grams

INGREDIENTS:

- 1 (8-ounce) package tempeh, crumbled
- 1/4 cup soy sauce
- 1 tablespoon maple syrup
- 1 tablespoon liquid smoke
- 1 teaspoon smoked paprika
- 1/2 teaspoon black pepper

INSTRUCTIONS:

1. Preheat oven to 375 degrees F (190 degrees C).
2. In a large bowl, mix the crumbled tempeh, soy sauce, maple syrup, liquid smoke, smoked paprika, and black pepper.
3. Toss to coat evenly.
4. Spread the tempeh in a single layer on a baking sheet.
5. Bake for 15 minutes, or until the tempeh is crispy.
6. Serve the tempeh "bacon" on its own or as a topping for salads, sandwiches, or wraps.

Tips:

1. For a hotter "bacon," add a pinch of cayenne pepper.
2. You may also add additional spices to the "bacon," such as cumin or coriander.

3. Store the tempeh "bacon" in an airtight jar in the refrigerator for up to 3 days.

DATE CARAMEL SAUCE

- Prep time: 10 minutes
- Cook time: 20 minutes
- Total time: 30 minutes

NUTRITIONAL DATA PER 1/4 CUP (60 GRAMS):

- Calories: 200
- Fat: 10 grams
- Protein: 2 grams
- Carbohydrates: 30 grams
- Fiber: 5 grams

INGREDIENTS:

- 1 cup (200 grams) pitted Medjool dates
- 1/2 cup (120 ml) unsweetened almond milk
- 1/4 cup (60 ml) water
- 1 tablespoon vanilla extract
- 1/4 teaspoon salt

INSTRUCTIONS:

1. In a food processor, blend the pitted dates, almond milk, water, vanilla essence, and salt.
2. Process until smooth and creamy.

3. If the sauce is too thick, add additional almond milk or water, 1 spoonful at a time.

4. If the sauce is too thin, simmer it over low heat until it thickens.

5. Taste and adjust spices as desired.

6. Serve the date caramel sauce over ice cream, fruit, or yogurt.

Tips:

1. For a thicker sauce, use full-fat coconut milk instead of almond milk.

2. You may also add additional spices to the sauce, such as cinnamon or nutmeg.

3. Store the date caramel sauce in an airtight jar in the refrigerator for up to 2 weeks.

ENCHILADA SAUCE

- **Prep time: 15 minutes**
- **Cook time: 20 minutes**
- **Total time: 35 minutes**

NUTRITIONAL DATA PER 1/4 CUP (60 GRAMS):

- Calories: 150
- Fat: 7 grams
- Protein: 3 grams
- Carbohydrates: 20 grams
- Fiber: 2 grams

INGREDIENTS:

- 1 tablespoon olive oil
- 1 onion, chopped
- 2 cloves garlic, minced
- 1 (14.5-ounce) can chopped tomatoes, undrained
- 1/2 cup tomato paste
- 1 tablespoon chili powder
- 1 teaspoon cumin powder
- 1/2 teaspoon dried oregano
- 1/4 teaspoon salt
- 1/4 teaspoon black pepper

INSTRUCTIONS:

1. In a large saucepan, heat the olive oil over medium heat.

2. Add the onion and simmer until softened, approximately 5 minutes.

3. Add the garlic and simmer for 1 minute longer, or until fragrant.

4. Add the chopped tomatoes, tomato paste, chili powder, cumin powder, dried oregano, salt, and pepper.

5. Bring to a boil, then decrease heat and simmer for 20 minutes, or until the sauce has thickened.

6. Taste and adjust spices as desired.

7. Serve the enchilada sauce over enchiladas, tacos, or burritos.

1. For a hotter enchilada sauce, add additional chili powder or cayenne pepper.
2. You may also add additional spices to the sauce, such as coriander or smoky paprika.
3. Store the enchilada sauce in an airtight jar in the refrigerator for up to 5 days.

FRESH BERRY AND MINT SALSA

- Prep time: 10 minutes
- Cook time: 0 minutes
- Total time: 10 minutes

NUTRITIONAL DATA PER 1/4 CUP (60 GRAMS):

- Calories: 50
- Fat: 1 gram
- Protein: 1 gram
- Carbohydrates: 12 grams
- Fiber: 2 grams

INGREDIENTS:

- 1 cup (150 grams) mixed berries
- 1/4 cup (15 grams) chopped fresh mint
- 1 tablespoon lime juice
- 1 tablespoon honey
- 1/4 teaspoon salt

INSTRUCTIONS:

1. In a small bowl, combine the mixed berries, chopped mint, lime juice, honey, and salt.
2. Toss to coat evenly.
3. Let the salsa rest for at least 15 minutes before serving to enable the flavors to blend.
4. Serve the fresh berry and mint salsa over grilled chicken, fish, or tofu.

Tips:

1. For a sweeter salsa, add extra honey.
2. You may also add additional berries to the salsa, such as raspberries or blueberries.
3. Store the fresh fruit and mint salsa in an airtight jar in the refrigerator for up to 3 days.

SUN-DRIED-TOMATO KETCHUP

- Prep time: 10 minutes
- Cook time: 15 minutes
- Total time: 25 minutes

NUTRITIONAL DATA PER 1/4 CUP (60 GRAMS):

- Calories: 100
- Fat: 5 grams

- Protein: 2 grams
- Carbohydrates: 15 grams
- Fiber: 1 gram

INGREDIENTS:

- 1/2 cup (75 grams) sun-dried tomatoes, packed in oil
- 1/4 cup (60 ml) tomato paste
- 1/4 cup (60 ml) apple cider vinegar
- 1 tablespoon lemon juice
- 1 tablespoon honey
- 1 teaspoon onion powder
- 1/2 teaspoon salt
- 1/4 teaspoon black pepper

INSTRUCTIONS:

1. In a food processor, blend the sun-dried tomatoes, tomato paste, apple cider vinegar, lemon juice, honey, onion powder, salt, and pepper.
2. Process until smooth and creamy.
3. Taste and adjust spices as desired.
4. Serve the sun-dried-tomato ketchup with hamburgers, fries, or sandwiches.

Tips:

1. For a hotter ketchup, add a sprinkle of cayenne pepper.
2. You may also add additional spices to the ketchup, such as paprika or cumin.

3. Store the sun-dried-tomato ketchup in an airtight jar in the refrigerator for up to 2 weeks.

SOUTHERN-STYLE REMOULADE SAUCE

- **Prep time: 15 minutes**
- **Cook time: 0 minutes**
- **Total time: 15 minutes**

NUTRITIONAL DATA PER 1/4 CUP (60 GRAMS):

- Calories: 200
- Fat: 15 grams
- Protein: 2 grams
- Carbohydrates: 15 grams
- Fiber: 1 gram

INGREDIENTS:

- 1/2 cup (120 ml) mayonnaise
- 1 tablespoon Dijon mustard
- 1 tablespoon Creole mustard
- 1 tablespoon lemon juice
- 1 tablespoon Worcestershire sauce
- 1 tablespoon capers, drained and rinsed
- 1 tablespoon chopped fresh parsley
- 1 tablespoon chopped fresh chives
- 1/2 teaspoon paprika
- 1/4 teaspoon salt

- 1/4 teaspoon black pepper

INSTRUCTIONS:

1. In a small bowl, mix together the mayonnaise, Dijon mustard, Creole mustard, lemon juice, Worcestershire sauce, capers, parsley, chives, paprika, salt, and pepper.
2. Taste and adjust spices as desired.
3. Serve the Southern-style remoulade sauce with fried seafood, po'boys, or shrimp and grits.

Tips:

1. For a hotter remoulade sauce, add a sprinkle of cayenne pepper.
2. You may also add additional herbs and spices to the sauce, such as thyme or celery seed.
3. Store the Southern-style remoulade sauce in an airtight jar in the refrigerator for up to 5 days.

HOMEMADE NONDAIRY, GLUTEN-FREE MILK

- **Prep time: 10 minutes**
- **Cook time: 0 minutes**
- **Total time: 10 minutes**

NUTRITIONAL VALUES FOR 1 CUP (240 ML):

- Calories: 100
- Fat: 5 grams
- Protein: 2 grams
- Carbohydrates: 15 grams
- Fiber: 1 gram

INGREDIENTS:

- 1 cup (100 grams) almonds
- 3 cups (720 ml) water

INSTRUCTIONS:

1. In a blender or food processor, mix the almonds and water.
2. Blend until smooth and creamy.
3. Strain the almond milk through a fine-mesh filter into a large basin.
4. Discard the solids.
5. Taste and adjust spices as desired.
6. Serve the homemade nondairy, gluten-free milk on cereal, in smoothies, or in baking.

Tips:

1. For a fuller milk, use full-fat coconut milk instead of water.
2. You may also add additional nuts to the milk, such as cashews or walnuts.
3. Store the homemade nondairy, gluten-free milk in an airtight container in the refrigerator for up to 3 days.

BUFFALO SAUCE

- Prep time: 5 minutes
- Cook time: 0 minutes
- Total time: 5 minutes

NUTRITIONAL DATA PER 1/4 CUP (60 GRAMS):

- Calories: 100
- Fat: 5 grams
- Protein: 1 gram
- Carbohydrates: 15 grams
- Fiber: 1 gram

INGREDIENTS:

- 1/2 cup (120 ml) spicy sauce
- 1/4 cup (60 ml) melted butter
- 2 tablespoons honey
- 1 tablespoon white vinegar
- 1 teaspoon cayenne pepper
- 1/2 teaspoon salt

INSTRUCTIONS:

1. In a small bowl, mix together the hot sauce, melted butter, honey, white vinegar, cayenne pepper, and salt.
2. Taste and adjust spices as desired.
3. Serve the buffalo sauce with chicken wings, French fries, or veggies.

Tips:

1. For a hotter buffalo sauce, add additional cayenne pepper.
2. You may also add additional spices to the sauce, such as garlic powder or onion powder.
3. Store the buffalo sauce in an airtight jar in the refrigerator for up to 2 weeks.

MOJO SAUCE

- Prep time: 10 minutes
- Cook time: 0 minutes
- Total time: 10 minutes

NUTRITIONAL DATA PER 1/4 CUP (60 GRAMS):

- Calories: 100
- Fat: 5 grams
- Protein: 1 gram
- Carbohydrates: 15 grams
- Fiber: 1 gram

INGREDIENTS:

- 1/4 cup (60 ml) olive oil
- 2 teaspoons lime juice
- 1 tablespoon chopped fresh cilantro
- 1 clove garlic, minced
- 1/2 teaspoon cumin powder
- 1/4 teaspoon salt
- 1/4 teaspoon black pepper

1. In a small bowl, mix together the olive oil, lime juice, cilantro, garlic, cumin powder, salt, and pepper.

2. Taste and adjust spices as desired.

3. Serve the mojo sauce over grilled chicken, fish, or vegetables.

1. For a hotter mojo sauce, add a sprinkle of cayenne pepper.

2. You may also add additional spices to the sauce, such as oregano or smoky paprika.

3. Store the mojo sauce in an airtight jar in the refrigerator for up to 5 days.

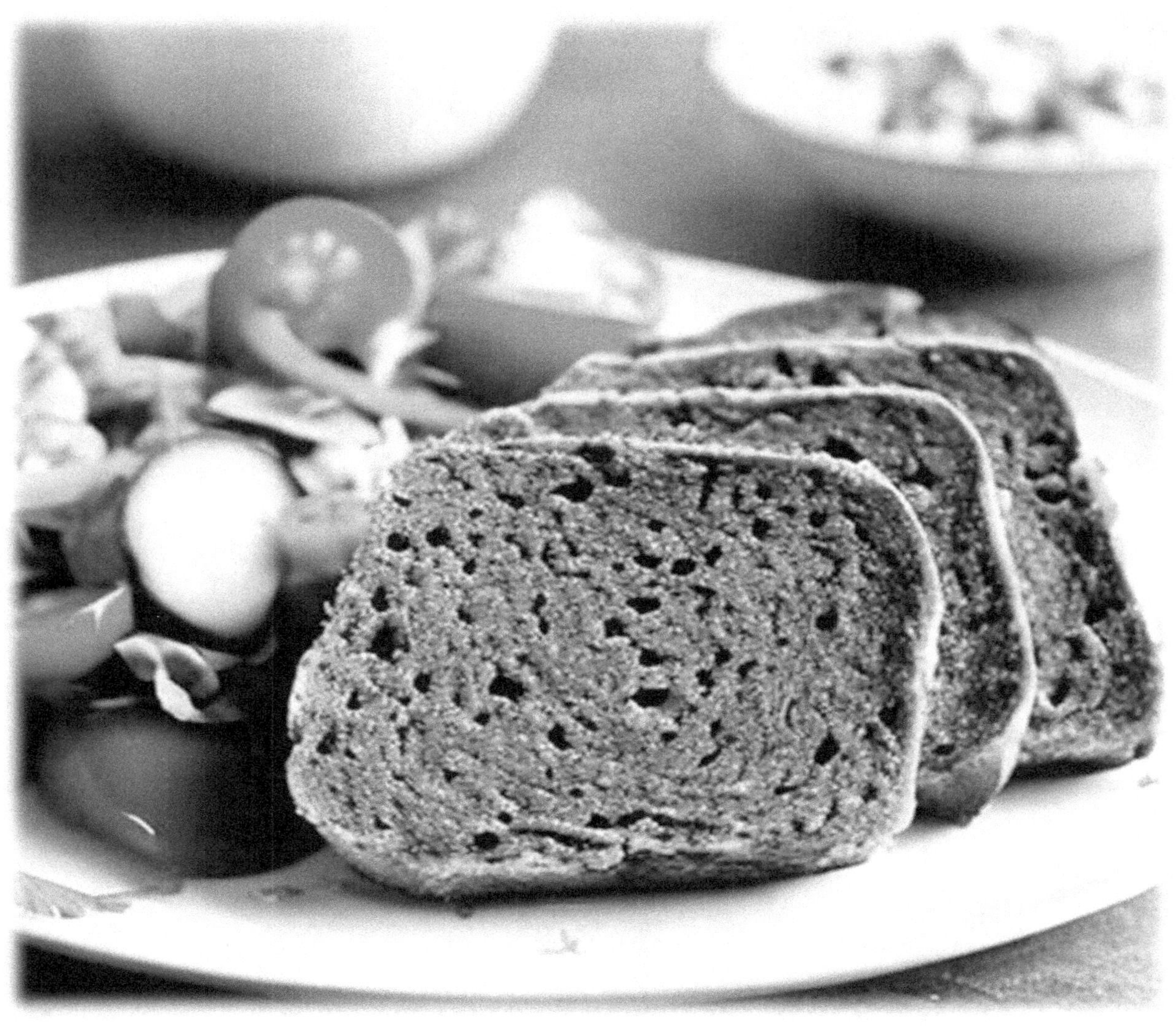

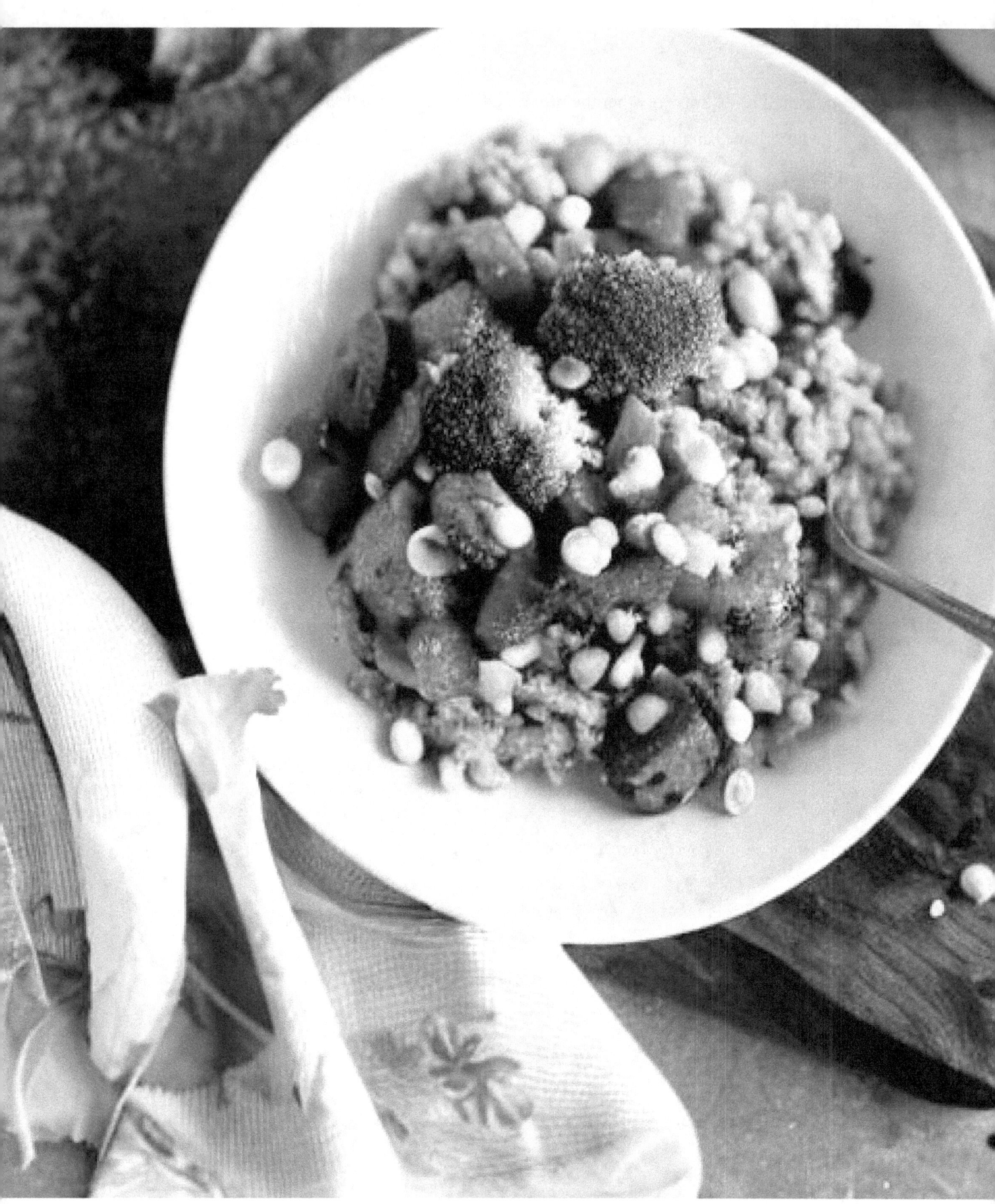

PECAN BARS

- **Prep time: 15 minutes**
- **Cooking time: 30 minutes**
- **Serving time: 10 minutes**
- **Total time: 55 minutes**

NUTRITIONAL VALUES PER SERVING:

- Calories: 300
- Fat: 18 grams
- Protein: 5 grams
- Carbohydrates: 35 grams
- Fiber: 5 grams

INGREDIENTS:

For the crust:

- 1 cup gluten-free all-purpose flour
- 1/2 cup almond flour
- 1/4 cup vegan butter, softened
- 1/4 cup powdered sugar
- 1/4 teaspoon salt

For the topping:

- 1 cup pecans, chopped
- 1/2 cup maple syrup
- 1/4 cup vegan butter
- 1/4 teaspoon cinnamon

INSTRUCTIONS:

1. Preheat oven to 350 degrees F (175 degrees C).
2. In a large bowl, mix the gluten-free flour, almond flour, vegan butter, powdered sugar, and salt.
3. Press the dough into an equal layer on the bottom of a greased 9x13 inch baking pan.
4. Bake for 15 minutes, or until the crust is softly golden brown.
5. In a small saucepan, mix the pecans, maple syrup, vegan butter, and cinnamon.
6. Cook over medium heat until the pecans are coated and the mixture is thickened, approximately 5 minutes.
7. Pour the pecan topping over the cooked crust.
8. Bake for 15 minutes longer, or until the topping is firm and bubbling.
9. Let the bars cool fully before cutting into squares.

Tips:

1. For a deeper taste, use dark maple syrup.

2. You may also add additional nuts or seeds to the topping, such as walnuts or sunflower seeds.

3. Store the Pecan Bars in an airtight jar at room temperature for up to 3 days.

AVOCADO BROWNIES

- Prep time: 10 minutes
- Cooking time: 20 minutes
- Serving time: 10 minutes
- Total time: 40 minutes

NUTRITIONAL VALUES PER SERVING:

- Calories: 250
- Fat: 15 grams
- Protein: 5 grams
- Carbohydrates: 30 grams
- Fiber: 5 grams

INGREDIENTS:

- 1 ripe avocado, mashed
- 1/2 cup unsweetened cocoa powder
- 1/2 cup maple syrup
- 1/4 cup almond flour
- 1/4 cup chopped dark chocolate
- 1 teaspoon vanilla extract
- 1/4 teaspoon salt

INSTRUCTIONS:

1. Preheat oven to 350 degrees F (175 degrees C).

2. Line an 8x8 inch baking tray with parchment paper.

3. In a large basin, mix the mashed avocado, cocoa powder, maple syrup, almond flour, chopped chocolate, vanilla essence, and salt.

4. Mix vigorously until the ingredients are uniformly distributed.

5. Pour the batter into the prepared baking pan.

6. Bake for 20 minutes, or until a toothpick inserted into the middle comes out clean.

7. Let the brownies cool fully before cutting into squares.

Tips:

1. For a deeper taste, use dark chocolate chips instead of chopped chocolate.

2. You may also add different toppings to the brownies, such as chopped nuts, coconut flakes, or chocolate icing.

3. Store the Avocado Brownies in an airtight jar in the refrigerator for up to 5 days.

APPLE CIDER MUFFINS

- Prep time: 15 minutes
- Cooking time: 20 minutes

Serving time: 10 minutes

Total time: 45 minutes

NUTRITIONAL VALUES PER SERVING:

- Calories: 200
- Fat: 10 grams
- Protein: 5 grams
- Carbohydrates: 30 grams
- Fiber: 4 grams

INGREDIENTS:

- 1 cup gluten-free all-purpose flour
- 1/2 cup almond flour
- 1/2 cup unsweetened applesauce
- 1/4 cup maple syrup
- 1/4 cup apple cider
- 1 tablespoon apple cider vinegar
- 1 teaspoon cinnamon
- 1/2 teaspoon nutmeg
- 1/4 teaspoon salt
- 1/2 cup chopped walnuts or pecans (optional)

INSTRUCTIONS:

1. Preheat oven to 375 degrees F (190 degrees C).
2. Line a muffin tin with paper liners or oil the cups with vegan butter.
3. In a large bowl, mix together the gluten-free flour, almond flour, cinnamon, nutmeg, and salt.
4. In a second dish, mix together the unsweetened applesauce, maple syrup, apple cider, apple cider vinegar, and chopped walnuts or pecans (if using).
5. Pour the wet ingredients into the dry ingredients and whisk until just incorporated.
6. Do not overmix.
7. Divide the batter equally among the muffin cups.
8. Bake for 20-25 minutes, or until a toothpick inserted into the middle of a muffin comes out clean.
9. Let the muffins cool in the muffin tin for 5 minutes before transferring them to a wire rack to cool fully.

Tips:

1. For a sweeter muffin, add one additional tablespoon of maple syrup.
2. You may also add additional spices to the muffins, such as ginger or cloves.
3. Store the Apple Cider Muffins in an airtight container at room temperature for up to 3 days.

DROP BISCUITS

Prep time: 10 minutes

- 🌰 Cooking time: 15 minutes
- 🌰 Serving time: 10 minutes
- 🌰 Total time: 35 minutes

NUTRITIONAL VALUES PER SERVING:

- 🌰 Calories: 150
- 🌰 Fat: 10 grams
- 🌰 Protein: 5 grams
- 🌰 Carbohydrates: 20 grams
- 🌰 Fiber: 2 grams

INGREDIENTS:

- 🌰 1 cup gluten-free all-purpose flour
- 🌰 1 tablespoon baking powder
- 🌰 1/2 teaspoon salt
- 🌰 1/4 cup vegan butter, softened
- 🌰 1/2 cup unsweetened almond milk

INSTRUCTIONS:

1. Preheat oven to 400 degrees F (200 degrees C)
2. Line a baking sheet with parchment paper.
3. In a large bowl, mix together the gluten-free flour, baking powder, and salt.
4. Cut in the vegan butter until the mixture resembles coarse crumbs.
5. Gradually add the almond milk, stirring until the dough barely comes together.
6. Drop the dough by rounded spoonful onto the prepared baking sheet.
7. Bake for 15-20 minutes, or until the biscuits are golden brown.
8. Let the biscuits cool on the baking pan for a few minutes before serving.

Tips:

1. For a fuller taste, use full-fat coconut milk instead of almond milk.
2. You may also add additional ingredients to the cookies, such as chopped herbs, shredded vegan cheese, or dried berries.
3. Store the Drop Biscuits in an airtight jar at room temperature for up to 2 days.

SALTED WALNUT-MAPLE BRITTLE

- 🌰 Prep time: 10 minutes
- 🌰 Cooking time: 15 minutes
- 🌰 Serving time: 5 minutes
- 🌰 Total time: 30 minutes

NUTRITIONAL VALUES PER SERVING:

- Calories: 200

- Fat: 12 grams

- Protein: 2 grams

- Carbohydrates: 28 grams

- Fiber: 1 gram

INGREDIENTS:

- 1 cup granulated sugar

- 1/2 cup maple syrup

- 1/4 cup vegan butter

- 1 cup chopped walnuts

- 1/2 teaspoon salt

INSTRUCTIONS:

1. Line a baking sheet with parchment paper.

2. In a medium saucepan, mix the granulated sugar, maple syrup, and vegan butter.

3. Cook over medium heat, stirring regularly, until the sugar is dissolved and the sauce is boiling.

4. Reduce the heat to low and continue to simmer for 5 minutes, or until the mixture is a rich caramel color.

5. Remove the pot from the heat and toss in the chopped walnuts and salt.

6. Pour the brittle onto the prepared baking sheet and distribute it evenly.

7. Let the brittle cool fully before breaking it into pieces.

1. For a hotter brittle, add a sprinkle of cayenne pepper to the recipe.

2. You may also add additional nuts or seeds to the brittle, such as pecans or sunflower seeds.

3. Store the Salted Walnut-Maple Brittle in an airtight jar at room temperature for up to 2 weeks.

MATCHA SHORTBREAD

- **Prep time: 15 minutes**

- **Cooking time: 20 minutes**

- **Serving time: 5 minutes**

- **Total time: 40 minutes**

NUTRITIONAL VALUES PER SERVING:

- Calories: 200

- Fat: 10 grams

- Protein: 2 grams

- Carbohydrates: 30 grams

- Fiber: 2 grams

INGREDIENTS:

- 1 cup vegan butter, softened

- 1/2 cup powdered sugar

- 1 cup gluten-free all-purpose flour

- 1 tablespoon matcha powder

- 1/4 teaspoon salt

1. Preheat oven to 350 degrees F (175 degrees C).
2. Line an 8x8 inch baking tray with parchment paper.
3. In a large bowl, mix together the vegan butter and powdered sugar until light and fluffy.
4. Gradually add the gluten-free flour, matcha powder, and salt, mixing until just incorporated.
5. Press the dough into the prepared baking pan.
6. Bake for 20-25 minutes, or until the edges are golden brown.
7. Let the shortbread cool fully in the pan before cutting into pieces.

Tips:

1. For a deeper taste, use full-fat vegan butter.
2. You may also add different flavorings to the shortbread, such as vanilla extract or almond extract.
3. Store the Matcha Shortbread in an airtight container at room temperature for up to 3 days

PEACH AND BLUEBERRY GALETTE

- Prep time: 20 minutes
- Cooking time: 30 minutes
- Serving time: 10 minutes
- Total time: 60 minutes

NUTRITIONAL VALUES PER SERVING:

- Calories: 250
- Fat: 15 grams
- Protein: 5 grams
- Carbohydrates: 30 grams
- Fiber: 3 grams

INGREDIENTS:

For the crust:

- 1 cup gluten-free all-purpose flour
- 1/4 cup vegan butter, softened
- 1/4 cup powdered sugar
- 1/4 teaspoon salt
- 2 tablespoons ice water

For the filling:

- 2 cups sliced peaches
- 1 cup blueberries
- 1/4 cup maple syrup
- 1 tablespoon lemon juice
- 1 teaspoon cornstarch

1. Preheat oven to 400 degrees F (200 degrees C).

2. In a large bowl, mix together the gluten-free flour, vegan butter, powdered sugar, and salt.

3. Gradually add the ice water, mixing until the dough barely comes together.

4. Form the dough into a disk, cover it in plastic wrap, and chill for 30 minutes.

5. On a lightly floured board, lay out the dough into a 12-inch circle.

6. Transfer the dough to a prepared baking sheet.

7. In a medium bowl, whisk together the sliced peaches, blueberries, maple syrup, lemon juice, and cornstarch.

8. Mound the peach-blueberry mixture in the middle of the dough, leaving a 2-inch border around the perimeter.

9. Fold the edges of the dough over the filling, pleating as desired.

10. Bake for 30-35 minutes, or until the crust is golden brown and the filling is bubbling.

11. Let the galette cool for 10 minutes before serving.

Tips:

1. For a sweeter galette, add one additional tablespoon of maple syrup.

2. You may also add additional fruits to the galette, such as plums or nectarines.

3. Store the Peach and Blueberry Galette in an airtight container at room temperature for up to 2 days.

SNICKERDOODLE BUNDT CAKE

- Prep time: 15 minutes
- Cooking time: 45 minutes
- Serving time: 10 minutes
- Total time: 60 minutes

NUTRITIONAL VALUES PER SERVING:

- Calories: 350
- Fat: 18 grams
- Protein: 5 grams
- Carbohydrates: 45 grams
- Fiber: 2 grams

INGREDIENTS:

For the cake:

- 1 1/2 cups gluten-free all-purpose flour
- 1 1/2 cups granulated sugar
- 1 teaspoon baking powder
- 1/2 teaspoon baking soda
- 1/2 teaspoon salt
- 1/2 cup vegan butter, softened

1 cup unsweetened almond milk

1 teaspoon vanilla extract

For the cinnamon-sugar topping:

1/4 cup granulated sugar

2 tablespoons ground cinnamon

INSTRUCTIONS:

1. Preheat oven to 350 degrees F (175 degrees C).
2. Grease and flour a 10-cup Bundt pan.
3. In a large bowl, mix together the gluten-free flour, granulated sugar, baking powder, baking soda, and salt.
4. In a separate dish, mix together the vegan butter, almond milk, and vanilla extract.
5. Gradually add the wet components to the dry ingredients, mixing until just incorporated.
6. Pour the batter into the prepared Bundt pan.
7. In a small bowl, mix the granulated sugar and cinnamon.
8. Sprinkle the cinnamon-sugar topping over the batter.
9. Bake for 45-50 minutes, or until a toothpick inserted into the middle comes out clean.
10. Let the cake sit in the pan for 10 minutes before transferring it onto a wire rack to cool fully.

Tips:

1. For a fuller taste, use full-fat coconut milk instead of almond milk.
2. You may also add additional spices to the cake mix, such as nutmeg or ginger.
3. Store the Snickerdoodle Bundt Cake in an airtight container at room temperature for up to 3 days.

NO-BAKE CARAMEL BROWNIE BARS

Prep time: 10 minutes

Cooking time: 2 hours

Serving time: 10 minutes

Total time: 2 hours 20 minutes

NUTRITIONAL VALUES PER SERVING:

Calories: 350

Fat: 20 grams

Protein: 5 grams

Carbohydrates: 35 grams

Fiber: 3 grams

INGREDIENTS:

For the brownie base:

- 1 cup gluten-free all-purpose flour
- 1/2 cup unsweetened cocoa powder
- 1/2 cup chopped nuts (such as almonds, walnuts, or pecans)
- 1/4 cup vegan butter, melted
- 1/4 cup maple syrup
- 1/4 cup unsweetened almond milk
- 1 teaspoon vanilla extract
- 1/4 teaspoon salt

For the caramel topping:

- 1 1/2 cups packed light brown sugar
- 1/2 cup vegan butter, sliced into bits
- 1/4 cup heavy cream
- 1/4 cup maple syrup
- 1 teaspoon vanilla extract
- 1/4 teaspoon salt

INSTRUCTIONS:

1. Line a 9x13 inch baking pan with parchment paper.
2. In a large bowl, mix together the gluten-free flour, cocoa powder, and chopped nuts.
3. In a separate dish, mix together the melted vegan butter, maple syrup, almond milk, vanilla extract, and salt.
4. Pour the wet ingredients into the dry ingredients and whisk until just incorporated.
5. Press the dough evenly into the prepared baking pan.
6. In a medium saucepan, mix the brown sugar, vegan butter, heavy cream, maple syrup, vanilla extract, and salt.
7. Cook over medium heat, stirring regularly, until the sugar is dissolved and the liquid is smooth and frothy.
8. Pour the caramel topping over the brownie foundation.
9. Refrigerate for at least 2 hours, or until the caramel has firm.
10. Cut the bars into squares and enjoy!

Tips:

1. For a fuller taste, use full-fat coconut milk instead of almond milk.
2. You may also add different toppings to the bars, such as chopped chocolate or sprinkles.
3. Store the No-Bake Caramel Brownie Bars in an airtight container in the refrigerator for up to 5 days.

ORANGE-VANILLA POUND CAKE

- Prep time: 15 minutes
- Cooking time: 50 minutes
- Serving time: 10 minutes
- Total time: 75 minutes

- Calories: 300
- Fat: 15 grams
- Protein: 5 grams
- Carbohydrates: 35 grams
- Fiber: 2 grams

INGREDIENTS:

- 1 cup (2 sticks) vegan butter, softened
- 1 cup granulated sugar
- 1 teaspoon vanilla extract
- 2 big eggs
- 2 cups gluten-free all-purpose flour
- 1 tablespoon baking powder
- 1/2 teaspoon salt
- 1/2 cup orange juice
- Zest of 1 orange

INSTRUCTIONS:

1. Preheat oven to 350 degrees F (175 degrees C).
2. Grease and flour a 9x5 inch loaf pan.
3. In a large bowl, mix together the vegan butter and granulated sugar until light and fluffy.
4. Beat in the vanilla essence and eggs one at a time.
5. In a separate dish, mix together the gluten-free flour, baking powder, and salt.
6. Gradually add the dry ingredients to the wet components, alternating with the orange juice.
7. Stir in the orange zest until barely incorporated.
8. Pour the batter into the prepared loaf pan.
9. Bake for 50-60 minutes, or until a toothpick inserted into the middle comes out clean.
10. Let the cake sit in the pan for 10 minutes before transferring it onto a wire rack to cool fully.

Tips:

1. For a fuller taste, use full-fat coconut milk instead of almond milk.
2. You may also add additional spices to the cake dough, such as cardamom or nutmeg.
3. Store the Orange-Vanilla Pound Cake in an airtight container at room temperature for up to 3 days.

SEEDED SANDWICH BREAD

- **Prep time: 20 minutes**
- **Rising time: 1 hour**
- **Baking time: 35 minutes**
- **Cooking time: 1 hour**
- **Total time: 2 hours 55 minutes**

- Calories: 250
- Fat: 5 grams
- Protein: 10 grams
- Carbohydrates: 40 grams
- Fiber: 5 grams

INGREDIENTS:

- 1 cup gluten-free all-purpose flour
- 1 cup whole wheat flour
- 1 tablespoon baking powder
- 1 teaspoon salt
- 2 teaspoons chia seeds
- 2 teaspoons flaxseed meal
- 2 teaspoons sunflower seeds
- 1 cup unsweetened almond milk
- 1 tablespoon apple cider vinegar
- 1 tablespoon vegetable oil

INSTRUCTIONS:

1. In a large bowl, mix together the gluten-free flour, whole wheat flour, baking powder, and salt.
2. Stir in the chia seeds, flaxseed meal, and sunflower seeds.
3. In a separate dish, mix together the unsweetened almond milk, apple cider vinegar, and vegetable oil.
4. Gradually add the wet components to the dry ingredients, stirring until just blended.
5. The dough will be sticky.
6. Turn the dough onto a lightly floured surface and knead for 5 minutes, or until the dough is smooth and elastic.
7. area the dough in an oiled basin, cover it with plastic wrap, and let it rise in a warm area for 1 hour.
8. Preheat oven to 375 degrees F (190 degrees C).
9. Punch down the dough and form it into a loaf.
10. Place the loaves on a prepared baking sheet.
11. Bake for 35 minutes, or until the crust is golden brown and a toothpick inserted into the middle comes out clean.
12. Let the bread sit in the pan for 10 minutes before transferring it to a wire rack to cool entirely.

Tips:

1. For a chewier bread, bake it for an extra 5 minutes.
2. You may also add additional seeds to the bread, such as pumpkin seeds or sesame seeds.

3. Store the Seeded Sandwich Bread in an airtight container at room temperature for up to 3 days.

BURGER BUNS

- Prep time: 20 minutes
- Rising time: 1 hour
- Baking time: 15 minutes
- Cooking time: 1 hour
- Total time: 2 hours 35 minutes

NUTRITIONAL VALUES PER SERVING:

- Calories: 200
- Fat: 5 grams
- Protein: 10 grams
- Carbohydrates: 30 grams
- Fiber: 2 grams

INGREDIENTS:

- 1 1/2 cups gluten-free all-purpose flour
- 1 tablespoon baking powder
- 1/2 teaspoon salt
- 1/4 cup vegan butter, softened
- 1 cup unsweetened almond milk
- 1 tablespoon apple cider vinegar
- 1 tablespoon sesame seeds (optional)

INSTRUCTIONS:

1. In a large bowl, mix together the gluten-free flour, baking powder, and salt.
2. Cut in the vegan butter until the mixture resembles coarse crumbs.
3. In a separate dish, mix together the unsweetened almond milk and apple cider vinegar.
4. Gradually add the wet components to the dry ingredients, mixing until just incorporated.
5. Do not overmix.
6. Turn the dough onto a lightly floured surface and knead for 5 minutes, or until the dough is smooth and elastic.
7. area the dough in an oiled basin, cover it with plastic wrap, and let it rise in a warm area for 1 hour.
8. Preheat oven to 375 degrees F (190 degrees C).
9. Line a baking sheet with parchment paper.
10. Punch down the dough and divide it into 8 equal pieces.
11. Shape each piece into a bun.
12. Place the buns on the prepared baking sheet.
13. Brush the tops of the buns with a little vegan butter or almond milk.
14. Sprinkle with sesame seeds, if preferred.

15. Bake for 15-20 minutes, or until the buns are golden brown and a toothpick inserted into the middle comes out clean.

16. Let the buns set on the baking sheet for 5 minutes before moving them to a wire rack to cool fully.

1. For a chewier bun, bake it for an extra 5 minutes.

2. You may also add different toppings to the buns, such as poppy seeds or dry herbs.

3. Store the Burger Buns in an airtight container at room temperature for up to 2 days.

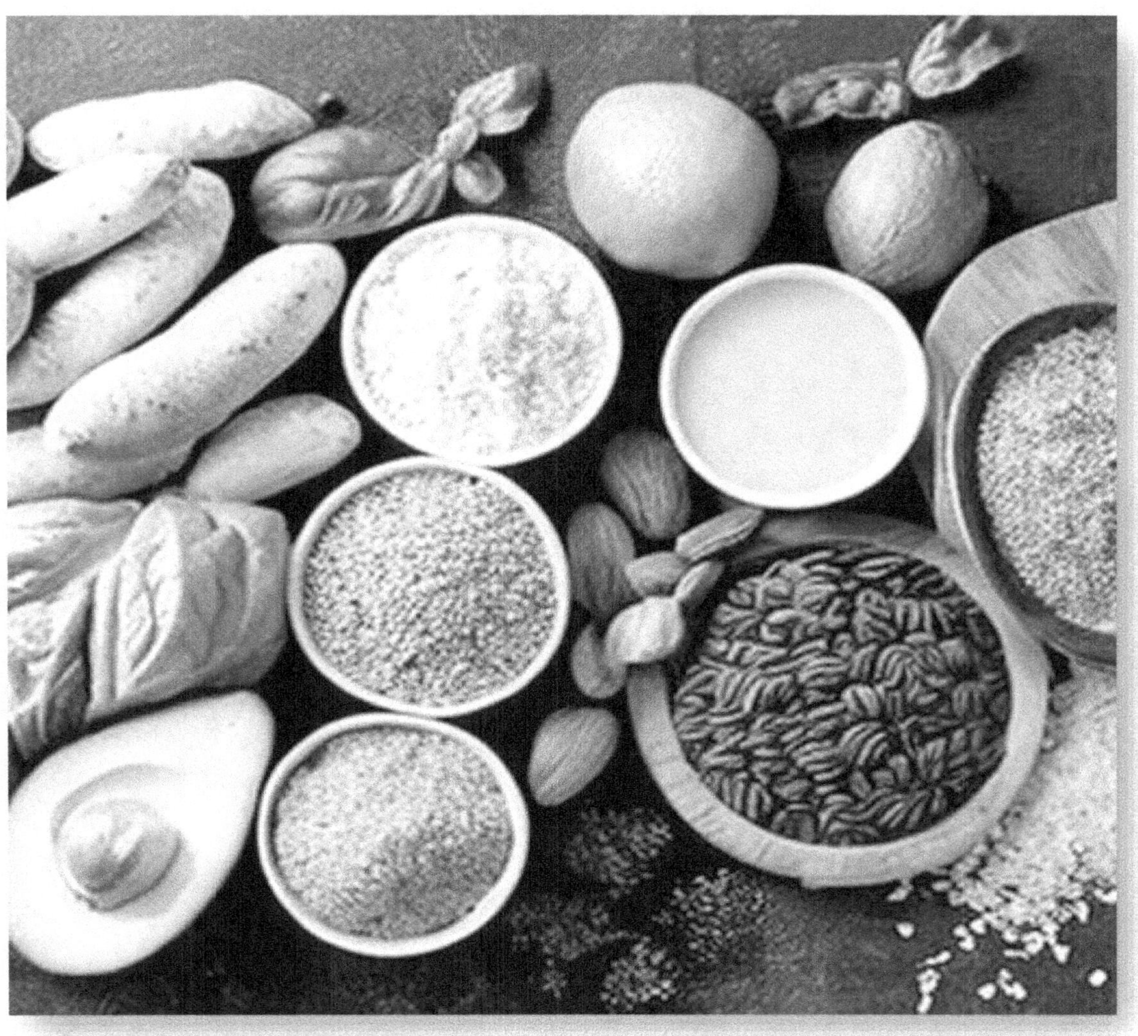

RECIPE CARD

Reciepe Card

COURSE: DIET: PREP TIME: COOK TIME: SERVINGS

INSTRUCTIONS

INGREDIENTS

Serves Prep Cook Time

TIPS & TRICKS

NOTES

Reciepe Card

COURSE:

DIET:

PREP TIME:

COOK TIME:

SERVINGS

INGREDIENTS

INSTRUCTIONS

Serves

Prep

Cook Time

TIPS & TRICKS

NOTES

Reciepe Card

COURSE:

DIET:

PREP TIME:

COOK TIME:

SERVINGS

INSTRUCTIONS

INGREDIENTS

Serves

Prep

Cook Time

TIPS & TRICKS

NOTES

Reciepe Card

INGREDIENTS

INSTRUCTIONS

Serves

Prep

Cook Time

TIPS & TRICKS

NOTES

Reciepe Card

COURSE: DIET: PREP TIME: COOK TIME: SERVINGS

INGREDIENTS

INSTRUCTIONS

Serves   Prep   Cook Time

TIPS & TRICKS

NOTES

Reciepe Card

COURSE:

DIET:

PREP TIME:

COOK TIME:

SERVINGS

INSTRUCTIONS

INGREDIENTS

Serves

Prep

Cook Time

TIPS & TRICKS

NOTES

Reciepe Card

COURSE:

DIET:

PREP TIME:

COOK TIME:

SERVINGS

INSTRUCTIONS

INGREDIENTS

Serves

Prep

Cook Time

TIPS & TRICKS

NOTES

Reciepe Card

COURSE: DIET: PREP TIME: COOK TIME: SERVINGS

INGREDIENTS

INSTRUCTIONS

Serves Prep Cook Time

TIPS & TRICKS

NOTES

Reciepe Card

COURSE: DIET: PREP TIME: COOK TIME: SERVINGS

INGREDIENTS

INSTRUCTIONS

Serves Prep Cook Time

TIPS & TRICKS

NOTES

Reciepe Card

INGREDIENTS

INSTRUCTIONS

Serves
Prep
Cook Time

TIPS & TRICKS

NOTES

Reciepe Card

COURSE: DIET: PREP TIME: COOK TIME: SERVINGS

INSTRUCTIONS

INGREDIENTS

Serves Prep Cook Time

TIPS & TRICKS

NOTES

Reciepe Card

COURSE:

DIET:

PREP TIME:

COOK TIME:

SERVINGS

INSTRUCTIONS

INGREDIENTS

Serves

Prep

Cook Time

TIPS & TRICKS

NOTES

Reciepe Card

COURSE:

DIET:

PREP TIME:

COOK TIME:

SERVINGS

INSTRUCTIONS

INGREDIENTS

Serves

Prep

Cook Time

TIPS & TRICKS

NOTES

Reciepe Card

COURSE: DIET: PREP TIME: COOK TIME: SERVINGS

INSTRUCTIONS

INGREDIENTS

Serves   Prep   Cook Time

TIPS & TRICKS

NOTES

Reciepe Card

COURSE: DIET: PREP TIME: COOK TIME: SERVINGS

INSTRUCTIONS

INGREDIENTS

Serves   Prep   Cook Time

TIPS & TRICKS

NOTES

Reciepe Card

INGREDIENTS

INSTRUCTIONS

TIPS & TRICKS

NOTES

Reciepe Card

COURSE:

DIET:

PREP TIME:

COOK TIME:

SERVINGS

INSTRUCTIONS

INGREDIENTS

Serves

Prep

Cook Time

TIPS & TRICKS

NOTES

Reciepe Card

COURSE: DIET: PREP TIME: COOK TIME: SERVINGS

INSTRUCTIONS

INGREDIENTS

Serves Prep Cook Time

TIPS & TRICKS

NOTES

Reciepe Card

COURSE:

DIET:

PREP TIME:

COOK TIME:

SERVINGS

INSTRUCTIONS

INGREDIENTS

Serves

Prep

Cook Time

TIPS & TRICKS

NOTES

Reciepe Card

COURSE: DIET: PREP TIME: COOK TIME: SERVINGS

INSTRUCTIONS

INGREDIENTS

Serves   Prep   Cook Time

TIPS & TRICKS

NOTES

Reciepe Card

COURSE: DIET: PREP TIME: COOK TIME: SERVINGS

INGREDIENTS

INSTRUCTIONS

Serves   Prep   Cook Time

TIPS & TRICKS

NOTES

Reciepe Card

COURSE:

DIET:

PREP TIME:

COOK TIME:

SERVINGS

INSTRUCTIONS

INGREDIENTS

Serves

Prep

Cook Time

TIPS & TRICKS

NOTES

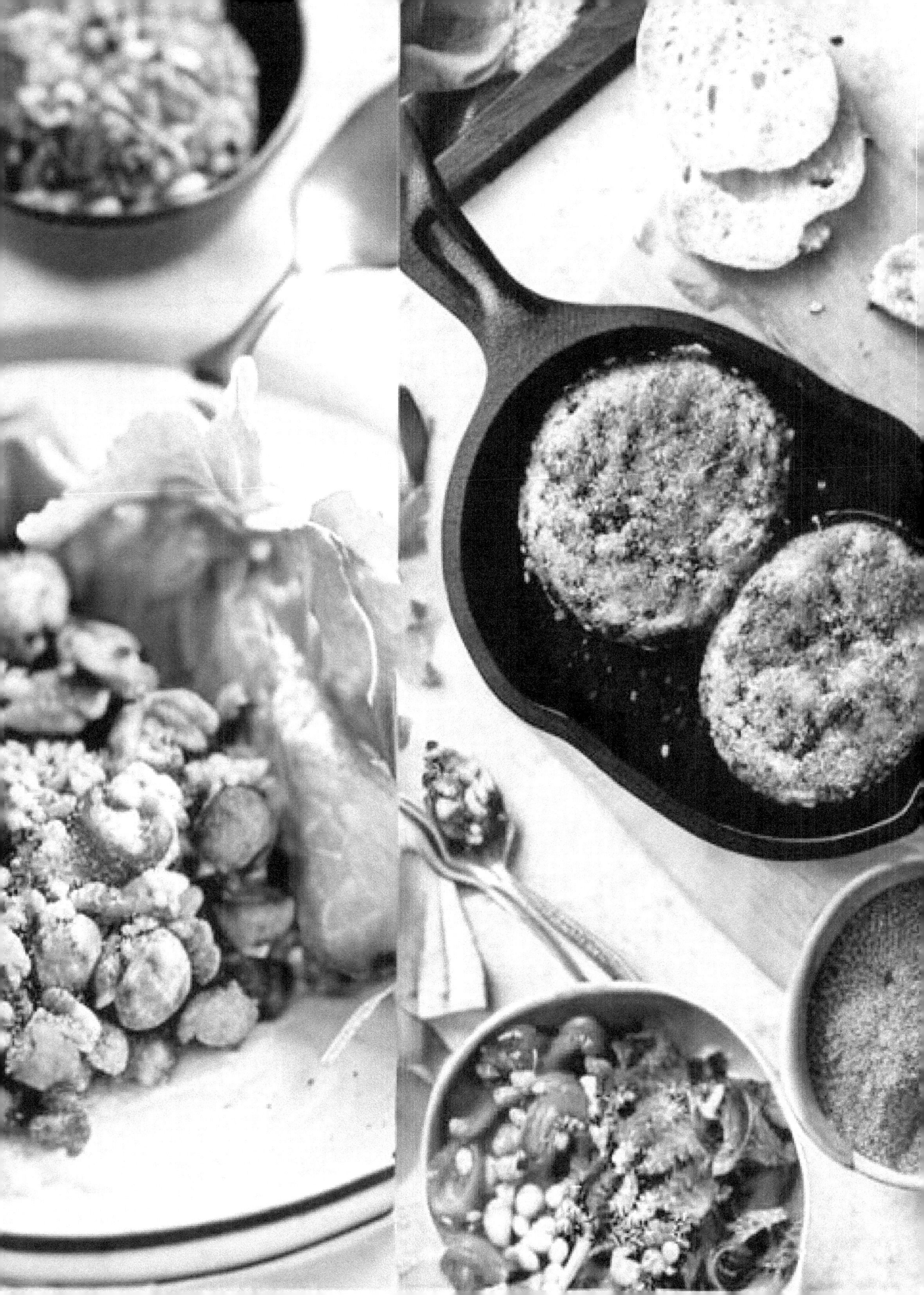